TO MY NIECE KIM
AND ALL THE
WORLD'S CHILDREN

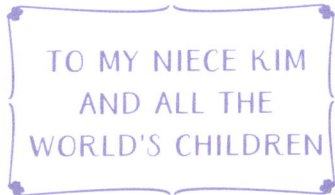

ISBN (HB) 978-4-8623907-3-8
ISBN (PB) 978-0-6450723-0-3
ISBN (E) 978-0-6450723-1-0

DISCLAIMER

Neither author nor publisher assume any responsibility for errors, inaccuracies, omissions, or any inconsistencies herein. The author and the publisher are not responsible for any adverse effects (injuries) or consequences resulting from the use of any of the poses and additional advice given in this book. Any use of the information set forth herein is entirely at the reader's discretion. Listen to your body and practice with an open mind and heart and you'll soon feel and reap the benefits of hatha yoga. As David Williams tells us: "Make yoga a 50-year goal, the turtle not the rabbit wins the race!"

PLEASE CONSIDER

The layout of this family yoga book is kid-friendly! As it is a book primarily geared at kids, text- heavy pages giving more in-depth understanding are at the back rather than the front of this book. Children aged 7 and younger will most likely want to get into doing the poses immediately and organically. Teachers, parents, educators and friends of children as well as older children please take note of the more intricate points as to why yoga is such a gift to humanity.

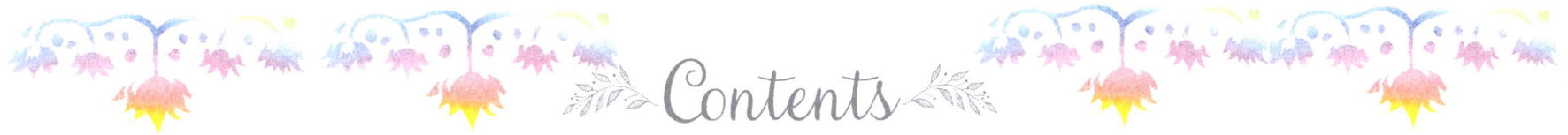

Contents

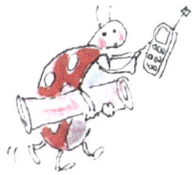
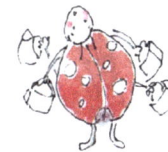
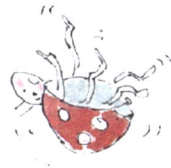
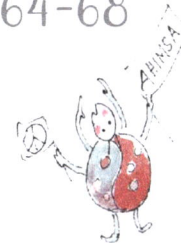
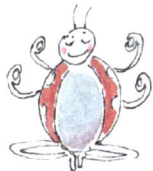
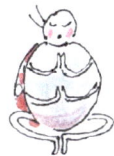
PARTIAL PROCEEDS OF SALES GO TO
DR JANE GOODALL'S ROOTS & SHOOTS NZ FOUNDATION AND TCHIMPOUNGA

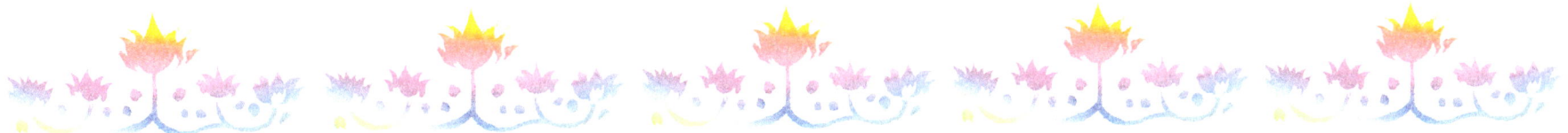

to everyone

One of the most mysterious things the ancient yogis understood is to respect nature. They even knew how to communicate with plants and animals. When a member in the community was sick, they understood the healing powers of plants and which plant would make the sick person better. They also had special yoga poses to help stay well or get well.

When you take care of your health by practicing yoga, you'll get to understand how important the environment is.

Many of the yoga poses in this book are named after animals, plants, warriors and natural monuments. Everything is connected. The sun is shining on the mountain, on the tree on the mountain, on the monkey on the tree, on the artist who is inspired by that monkey and brings him to you in the form of the character Aristotle.

Aristotle is here to teach you to take care of your body by letting it move freely, the way nature intended.

Even if there is no one around for you to do yoga with, remember you're not alone. You can join Aristotle and do yoga with him daily. It will keep your mind and body focused and healthy and your heart open and happy. Understand, everything is connected. We are not apart from but a part of our surroundings. Namaste, peace on earth.

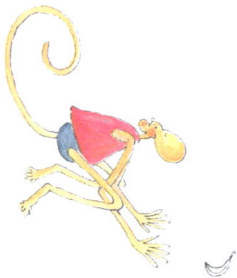

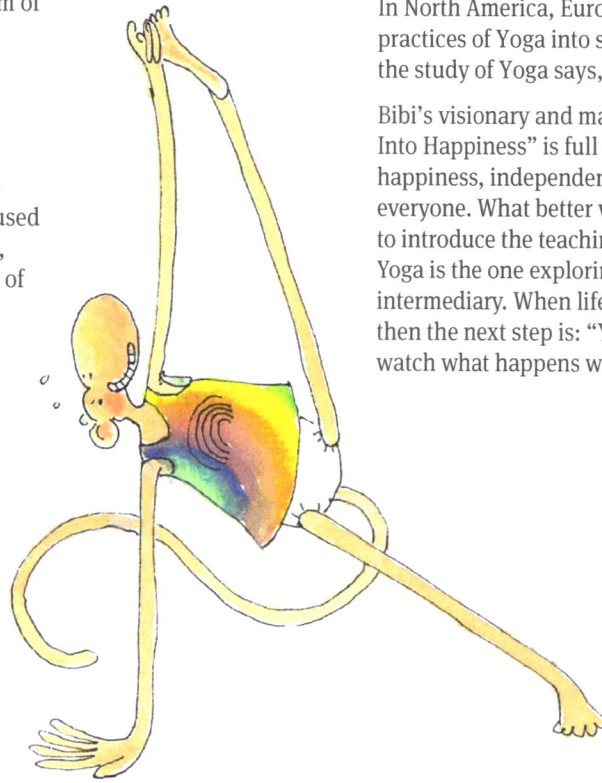

foreword from Danny Paradise

What is to be the future of the Earth?

What will be the legacy we leave our children?

The Native Americans say, "a Spiritual Warrior is someone who continuously creates a world of balance and harmony for coming generations."

In the last 30 years the teachings of Yoga have come to us in full force. An ancient wisdom and science that helps individuals fulfil their personal destiny . . . a foundation for living, for healing, for peace, for strength, balance, flexibility, evolution and for aging with vitality and grace. Krishnamacharya, the "Grandfather" of Yoga in the world, described the purpose of Yoga to be the creation of happiness in one's life.

In North America, Europe and Asia there are major movements to bring the practices of Yoga into school curriculums. Everyone I know who has begun the study of Yoga says, "I wish I had learned this when I was younger!"

Bibi's visionary and masterful new children's book "Aristotle's Journey Into Happiness" is full of ancient wisdom, beautiful drawings and the joy, happiness, independence and personal empowerment that Yoga can bring to everyone. What better way to help heal the world and restore the balance than to introduce the teachings of Yoga to the youngest generation? The Master of Yoga is the one exploring the evolutionary teachings . . . not the guru or the intermediary. When life force is abundant and consciousness is expanding then the next step is: "You've got to go where your heart says go . . . and then watch what happens when you follow your star!"

Danny Paradise April 2007
Molokai Hawaii International Yoga Instructor,
Song Writer, Musician, Film Maker.
www.dannyparadise.com

BEFORE ARISTOTLE THE
MONKEY MET DANNY
THE YOGI, HE OFTEN HAD
FALLING DREAMS.

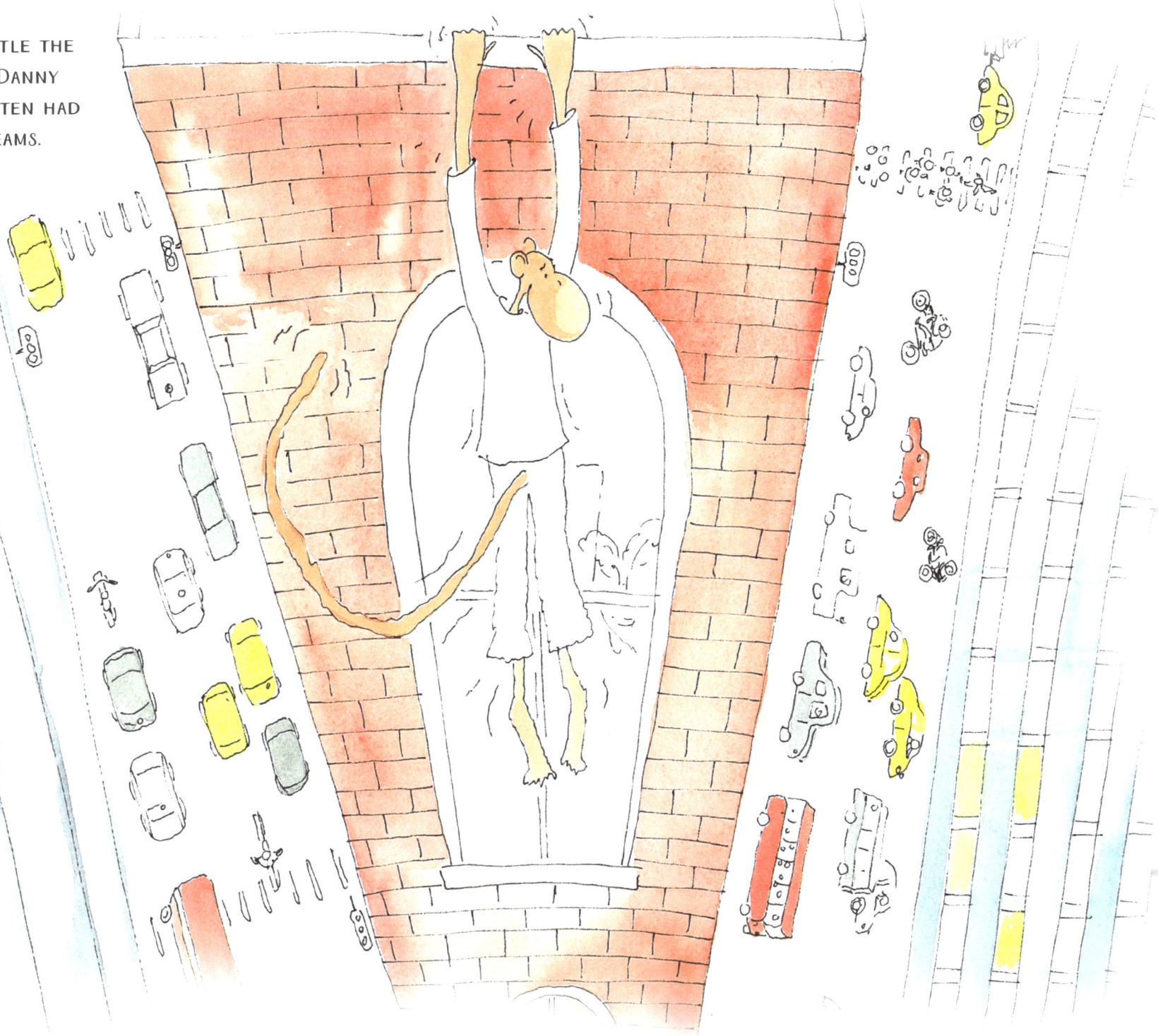

from breakdown to breakthrough

Not so long ago I was an easily distracted, overzealous and hyperactive, frazzled monkey. I jumped at anything that grabbed my curiosity. Sleeping was not my favourite pastime. I kept having nightmares of hanging off an extremely tall skyscraper about to topple off into the abyss. I never knew how to relax and enjoy the moment.

Then one day Danny came along, pulled out his shiny guitar and sang this song:

"Don't worry too much about who you are
tall, round, furry-tailed, near or far
what matters is that you follow your heart
the world is beautiful and she's all we've got.

It's ok to make mistakes
the mind opens up when the boundaries break
don't limit yourself to what you know or else
you'll never ever grow.

Don't worry too much about who you are
brown, patchy, bushy-haired, unknown or a star
what matters is that you listen to your heart
life is a gift so make the best of what you've got.

It's ok to say I'm scared
but try not let fear stop you, go follow the light
the lotus doesn't hide in the mud and dirt
she grows up to the sun where it's nice and bright.

Grow, follow that light, go follow your heart
fly high and smile with me. I'll never be far
I'll teach you to sing and a whole lot more
come be my friend, walk through that door."

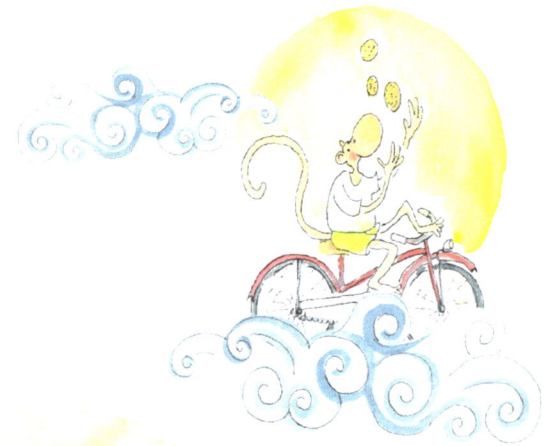

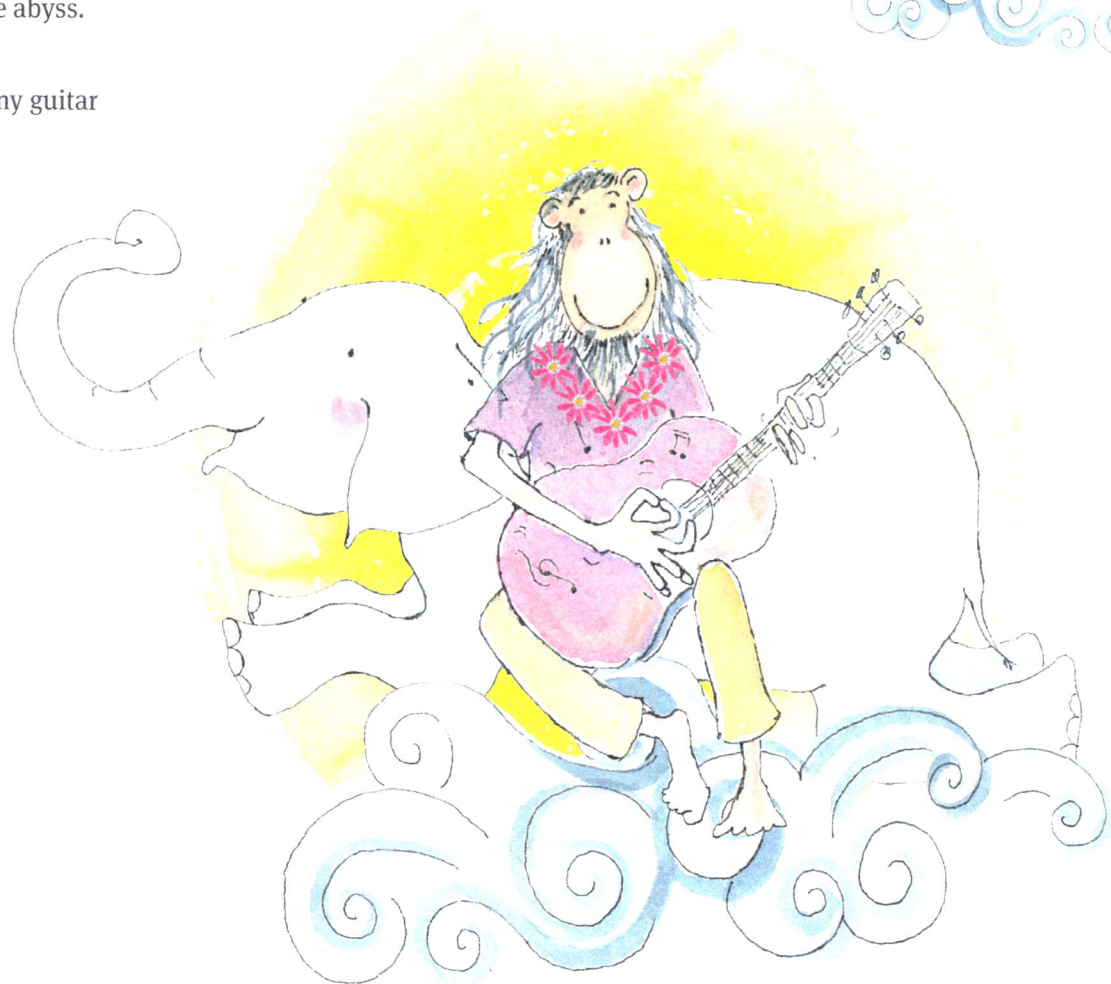

Then Danny dropped his guitar and jumped up into the most wonderful handstand with limbs and body twisted into all sorts of fantastic and breath-taking directions and shapes. I could hardly believe my eyes.

He played his body just like a musical instrument, plucking and stretching his every muscle like strings on a guitar. One moment his limbs soared high and gracefully like a bird and then they hovered light and low like a dragonfly above the watery surface, his breath dancing and vibrating to the tone of his entire being. This was fabulous...

From that day forward my life changed forever and continues to change in the most magical ways...and the best thing of all is that I made a true friend...so I say to you now:

"Grow, follow that light, go follow your heart, fly high and smile with me. I'll never be far I'll teach you to move and a whole lot more, come be my friend, walk through that door . . ."

OM, PEACE ON EARTH.

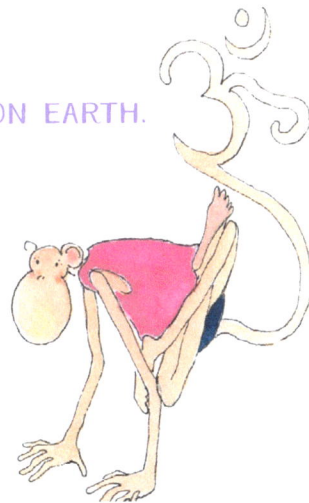

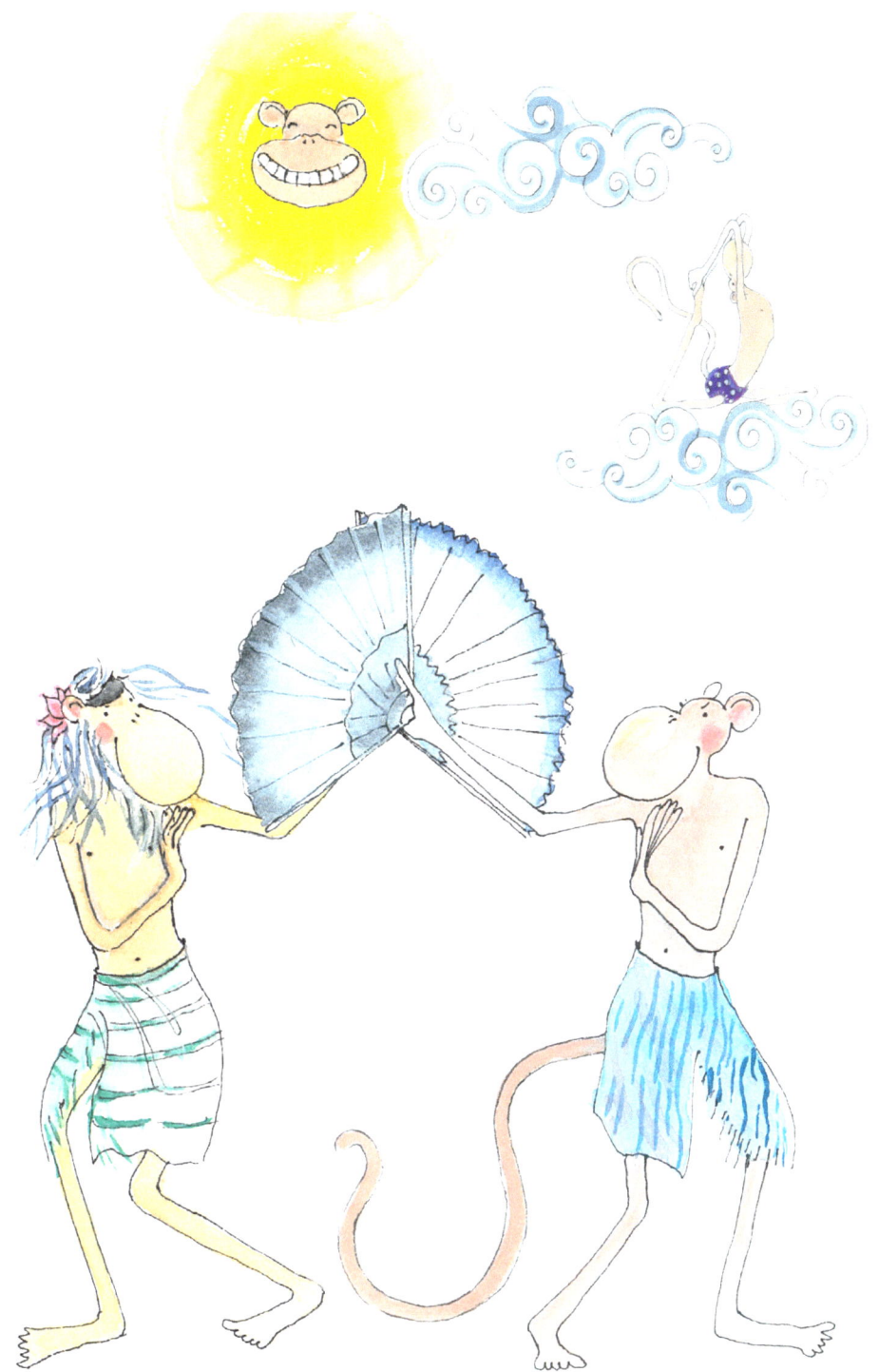

♡7♡

precautionary advice

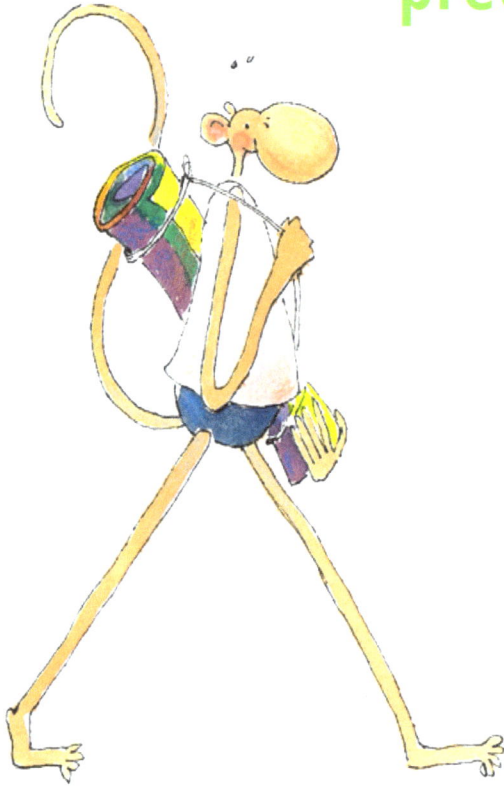

1 SMILE

Have fun and enjoy yoga, that is possibly the most important rule. A little bit every day goes a long way.

2 INJURIES

Make sure you have no old or new injuries. You don't want to re-injure yourself. If you're not sure, ask a wise teacher, a friend, someone in the family, a loved one or the doctor whether it's OK for you to do yoga. (Many doctors are now getting interested in the healing aspects of yoga). A skilled yoga teacher can also advise and will care about your wellbeing.

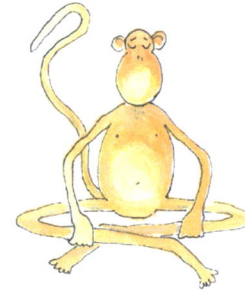

3 BARE FEET

Do yoga postures with bare feet to prevent slipping.

4 MAT

You'll want a mat or rug for comfort. If it's eco-friendly even better!

5 EMPTY STOMACH

Try not to eat a full meal for at least two hours before doing yoga. If you're really hungry and can't wait then eat a light snack, maybe a banana or apple, something which falls off a tree or bush or is pulled out of the soil (celery stick, or have carrot juice).

Natural, seasonal foods are best (if possible organic), lightly steamed or fresh.

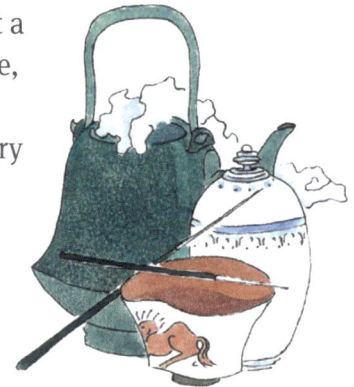

6   BE YOURSELF

Don't strive for some picture-perfect image you think yoga is! Start with yourself and remember, you're unique and wonderful just as you are now. Breathe, smile and listen to your body and mind. Remain comfortable in a posture.

7   PATIENCE, LOVE AND STAYING POWER

Even if you'll never be able to do a pose 'perfectly', patience, love and an ounce of staying power (also understood as faith/self-discipline) are the essence of your practice. Some monkeys start yoga at a very old age. Most likely they will not ever be able to do many of the poses, and that's OK. A wise monkey knows his/her physical limits and never tries to overdo it or show off.

If grandad does yoga with you he will want to use a chair. That's OK too.

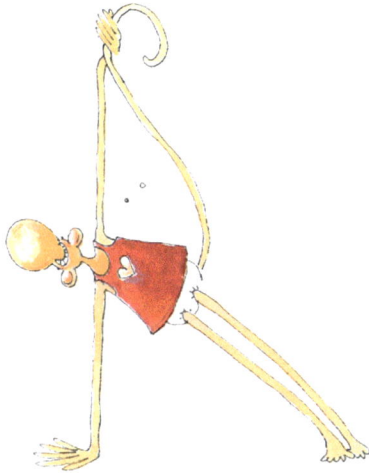

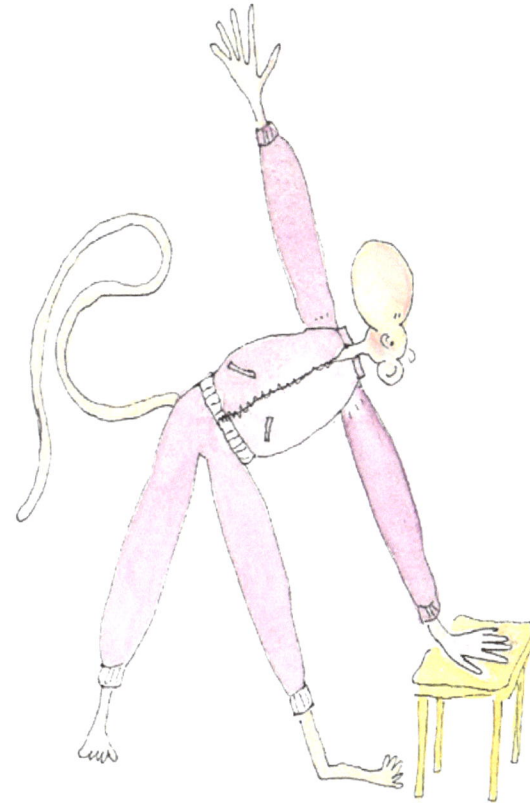

8   ALL IS ONE AND ONE IS ALL

Surround yourself with kind, honest, creative and natural friends. This is the 'Satsang of Yoga' and makes everyone feel supported, cheerful and positive. Beautiful minds make for beautiful bodies, lungs and hearts.

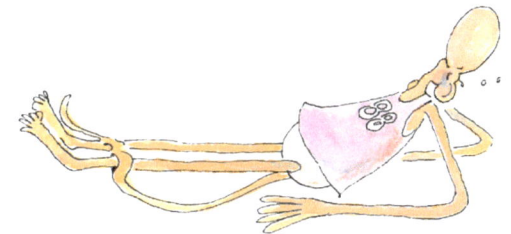

sitting quietly

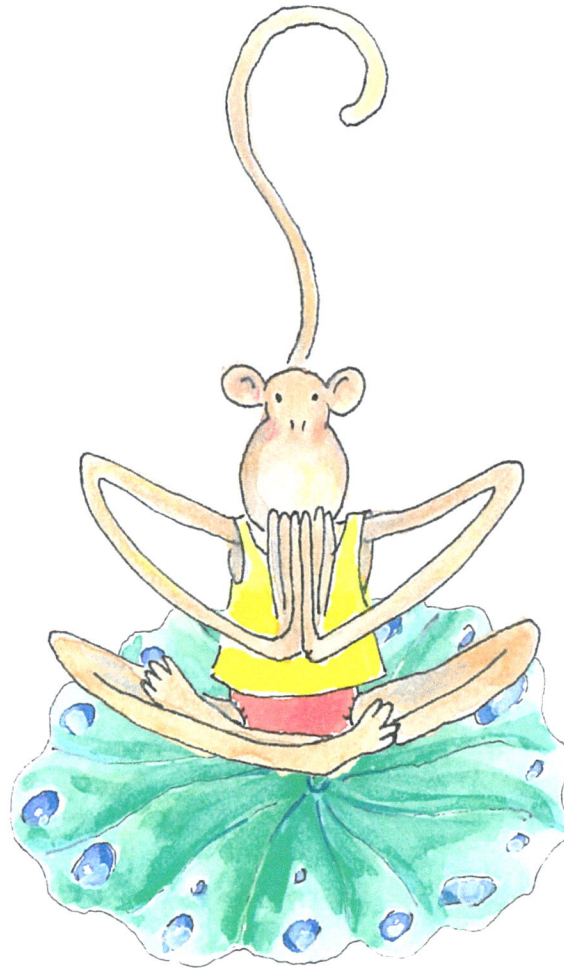

ZEN POINT

When the cow is thirsty she flicks her tail (the skilled whip). The sound makes the calf understand he needs to follow his mother to the river where they can drink.

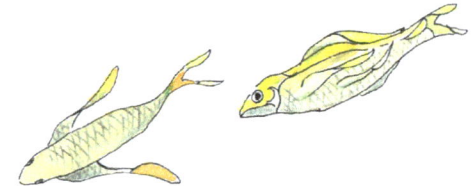

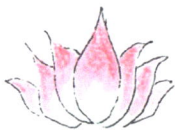

LEARNING TO LISTEN

Sit quietly in a comfortable position, a chair is also ok, with your back straight. Imagine the crown of your head being pulled up by an invisible string, bring your hands to your heart and breathe quietly. Let your thoughts drift by like clouds in the sky.

breathing

"WE SHOULD BEHAVE TO THE WORLD AS
WE WISH THE WORLD TO BEHAVE TO US."

- ARISTOTLE

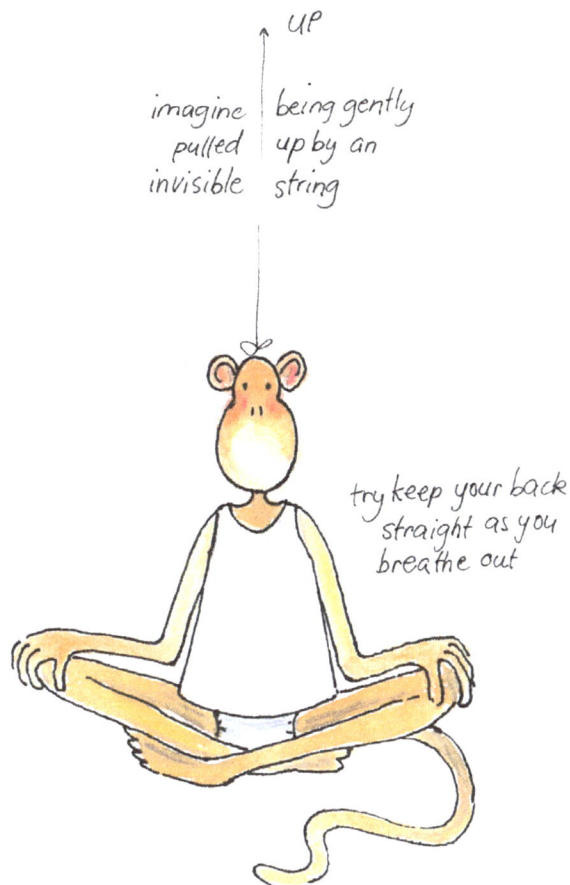

UP

imagine | being gently
pulled | up by an
invisible | string

try keep your back
straight as you
breathe out

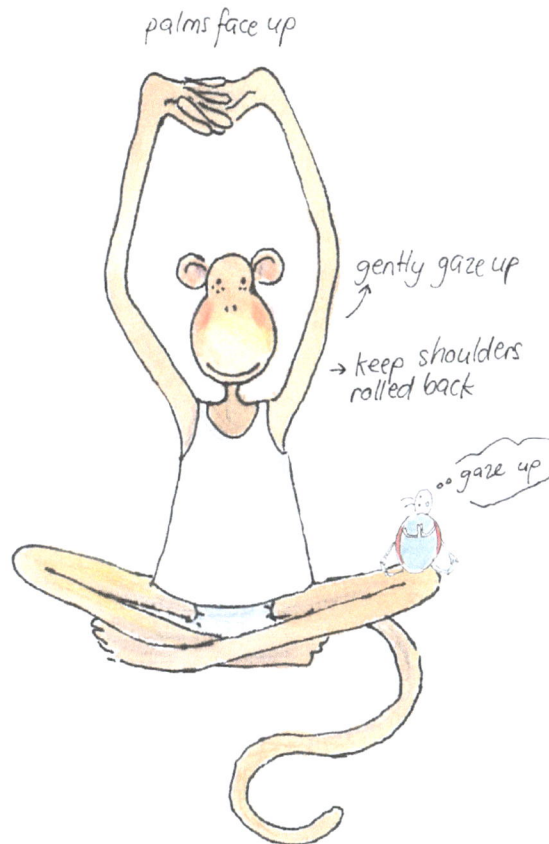

palms face up

gently gaze up

→ keep shoulders
rolled back

°° gaze up

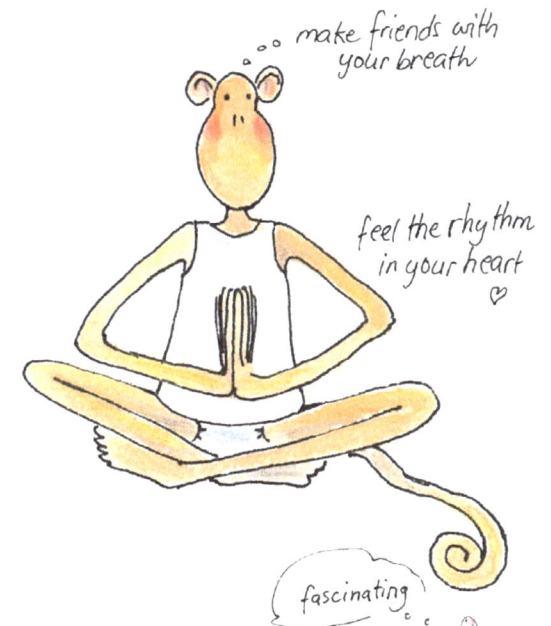

°° make friends with
your breath

feel the rhythm
in your heart ♡

fascinating

the lungs are very important
organs. The lungs and the
brain.

1

Sit cross-legged and breathe deeply in
and out through your nose. Don't rush the
breath, imagine it moves like the waves
coming in and out, to and from the shore.

2

Now interlock your fingers and stretch
your body and arms. Breathe a few times
in this position and lower your arms.
Repeat.

3

Watch how breath makes you feel
calmer. By Focusing on the breath
helps you stay present.

table-top refresher

This pose strengthens the arms, legs, hips, belly and back
and opens the chest for deeper breathing.

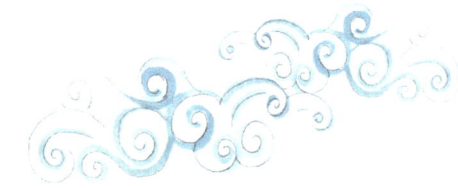

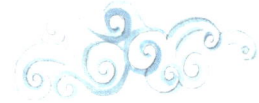

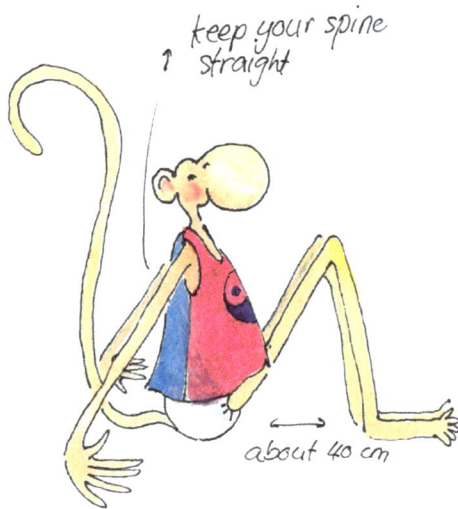

keep your spine straight

about 40 cm

the heart faces upward

shoulders are rolled back not slouched

lift the pelvis

knees above heels

smile and breathe

gently tilt

knees are hip-width apart

tailbone is tucked under

1

Sit on your bottom and tuck your knees in, hip width apart. Place your hands behind you, fingers pointing forward.

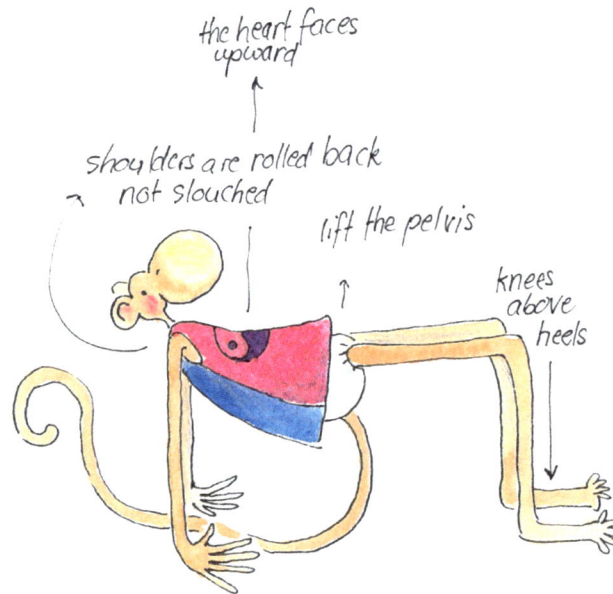

2

Press your palms and feet into the mat as you lift your pelvis. Keep your shoulders rolled back and the heart facing up.

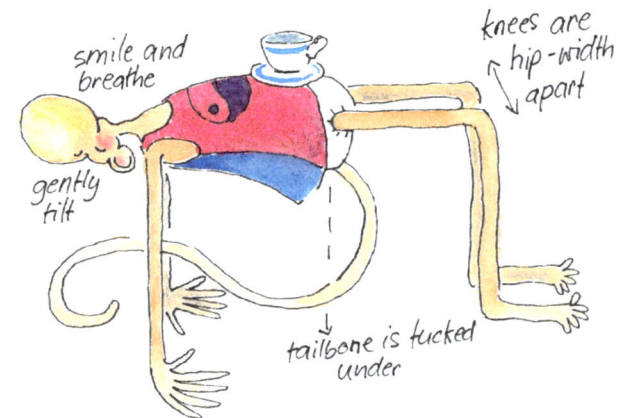

3

Carefully tilt your head back without hurting your neck. Stay in this pose for 10 counts and don't forget to breathe. Repeat steps 1 to 3 three times. Then slowly come down, lie back and give your knees a cuddle! Yummy!

back-roll refresher

This exercise is great for your lymphatic system and getting rid of tired energy and a cloggy mind.

If your back feels a bit bony, use a blanket on top of the mat to do this fun back roll.

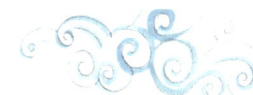

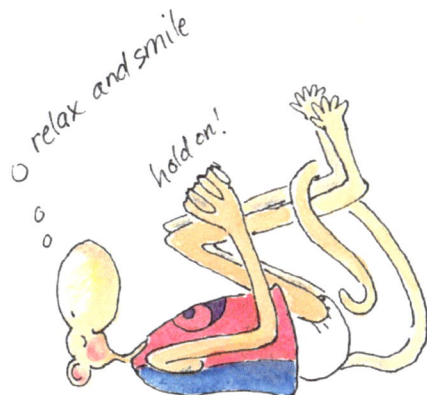

o relax and smile

hold on!

kick and roll

use two mats or a blanket if the floor is hard

monkeys need to stay mindful as to not roll onto their sensitive tails.

the tailbone is in the same place as in humans

1

Lie on your back with your knees tucked in and your hands clasped around your knees. Become aware of the space around you.

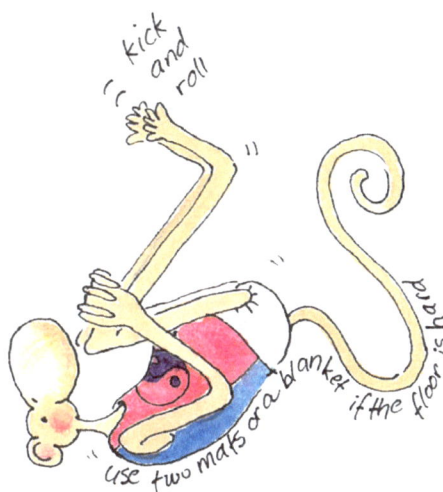

2

Kick-start the legs into a gentle back-rolling motion and smile as you do this.

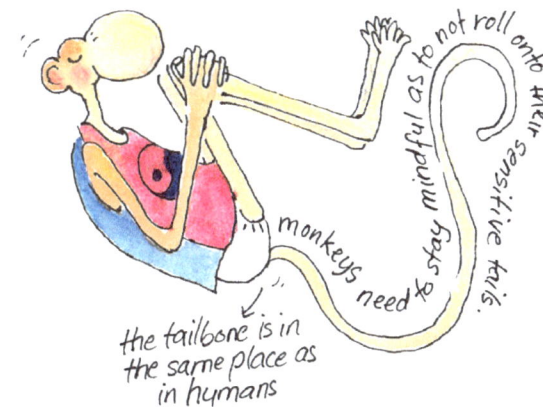

3

Swing back and forth at least ten times. Give your legs a good tuck each time. This is really fun and massages your back and shoulders. "Haaaaaa. Bliss!"

cat pose

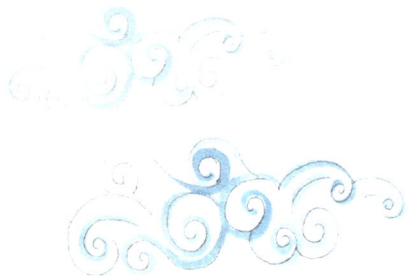

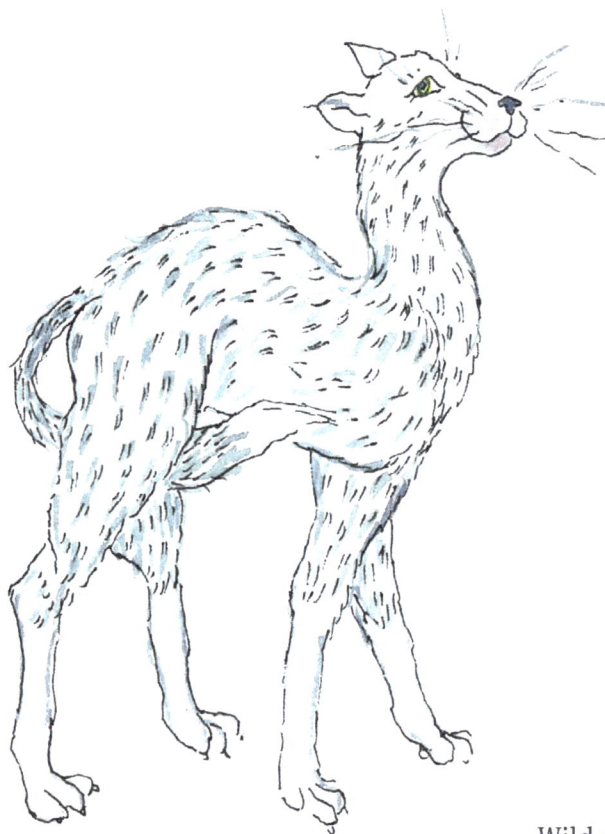

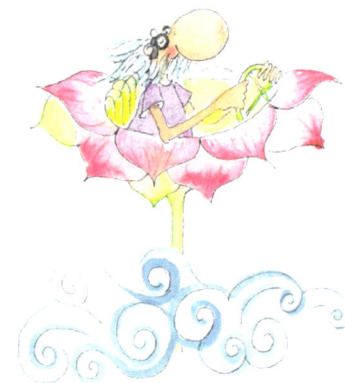

ZEN POINT

When the cat is happy she purrs, when angry she hisses. Observe how your breath changes depending on your mood. Learn to gauge your breath to balance your mood.

Speak your mind even if your voice shakes.

MINDFUL FACT

Wild cats walk long distances to catch their prey. Many house cats suffer from inactivity, weight problems and even stress, just like anyone who's not active enough.

Cat pose is a wonderful warm-up exercise for your spine. It brings fresh blood flow to the brain and strengthens and expands the lungs.

Coordinating and unifying breath with movement leads to a focused mind.

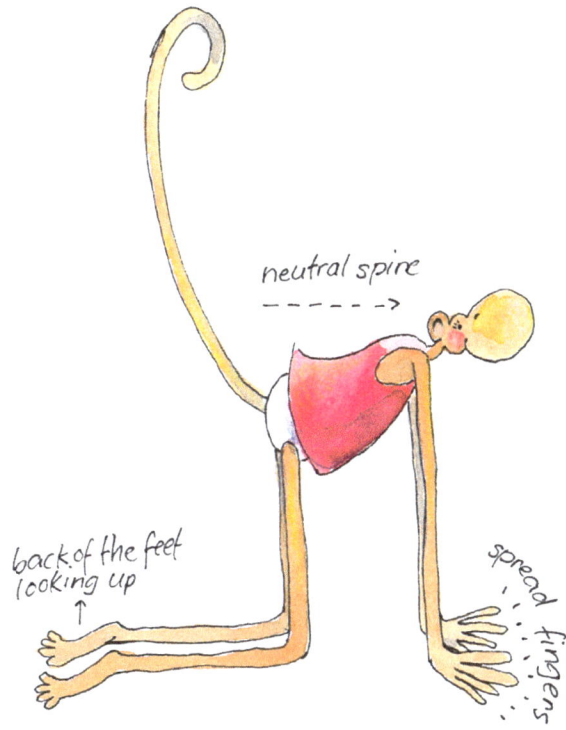

neutral spine
- - - - - →

back of the feet looking up
↑

spread fingers

Cat-Tilt—tuck the tailbone under

hands shoulder-width apart

knees hip-width apart

Dog-Tilt—tilt the tailbone up like a happy doggy

1

2

3

Bring your hands below your shoulders and your knees below your hips and relax.

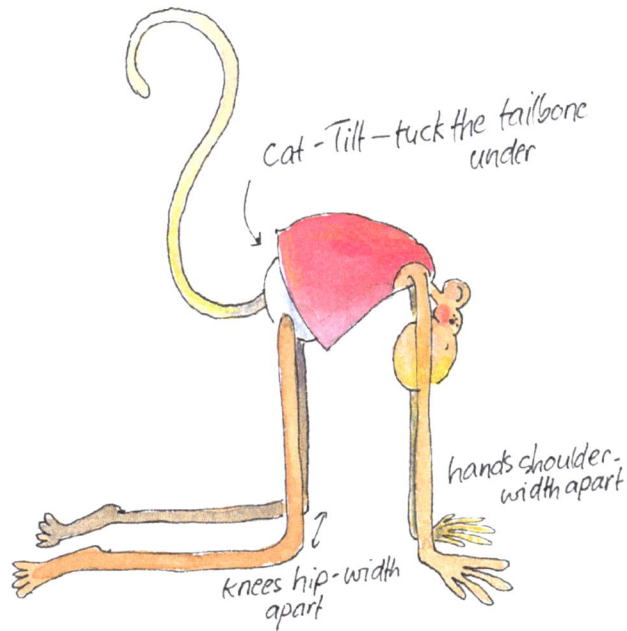

Breathe in, arch your back up and tuck your head and tailbone under.

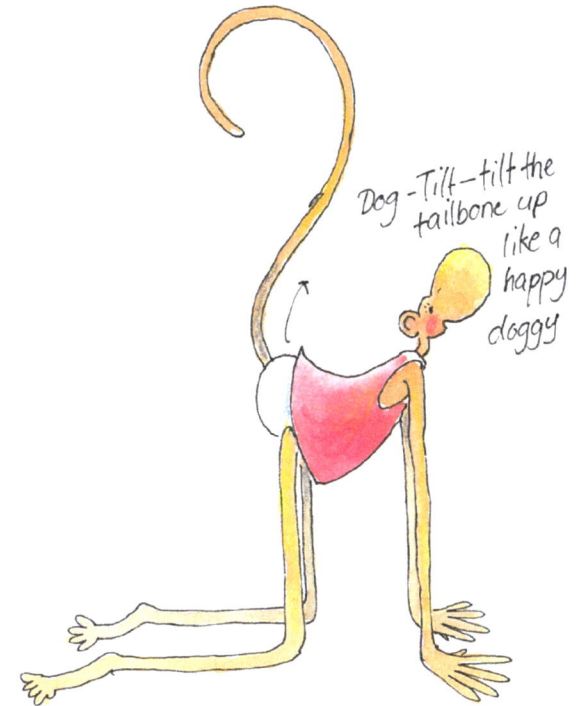

Breathe out, lower your spine and open your chest. Do numbers 2 and 3 six times.

child's pose

Resting poses help the body calm the mind and lower the heart rate.
Challenge yourself but also know when to rest.

ZEN POINT

TODAY, YOGA IS PRACTICED BY PEOPLE IN EVERY CORNER OF THE WORLD, FROM EVERY KIND OF BACKGROUND. SCHOOL CHILDREN AND CHILDREN WITH SPECIAL NEEDS, THE ELDERLY, STRESSED EXECUTIVES, PRISONERS, SICK PEOPLE, HEALTHY PEOPLE, ADDICTS IN RECOVERY, EXPECTANT MOTHERS, THE RICH AND THE POOR, CHRISTIANS, MUSLIMS, HINDUS, JEWS, BUDDHISTS, ETC. THEY ARE ALL PRACTISING YOGA, REAPING ITS BENEFITS IN ONE FORM OR ANOTHER. THIS WOULD HAVE BEEN INCONCEIVABLE TO A YOGI OR TO ANY INDIAN IN THE EARLY TWENTIETH CENTURY.

– KAUSTHUB DESIKARCHAR, THE YOGA OF THE YOGI

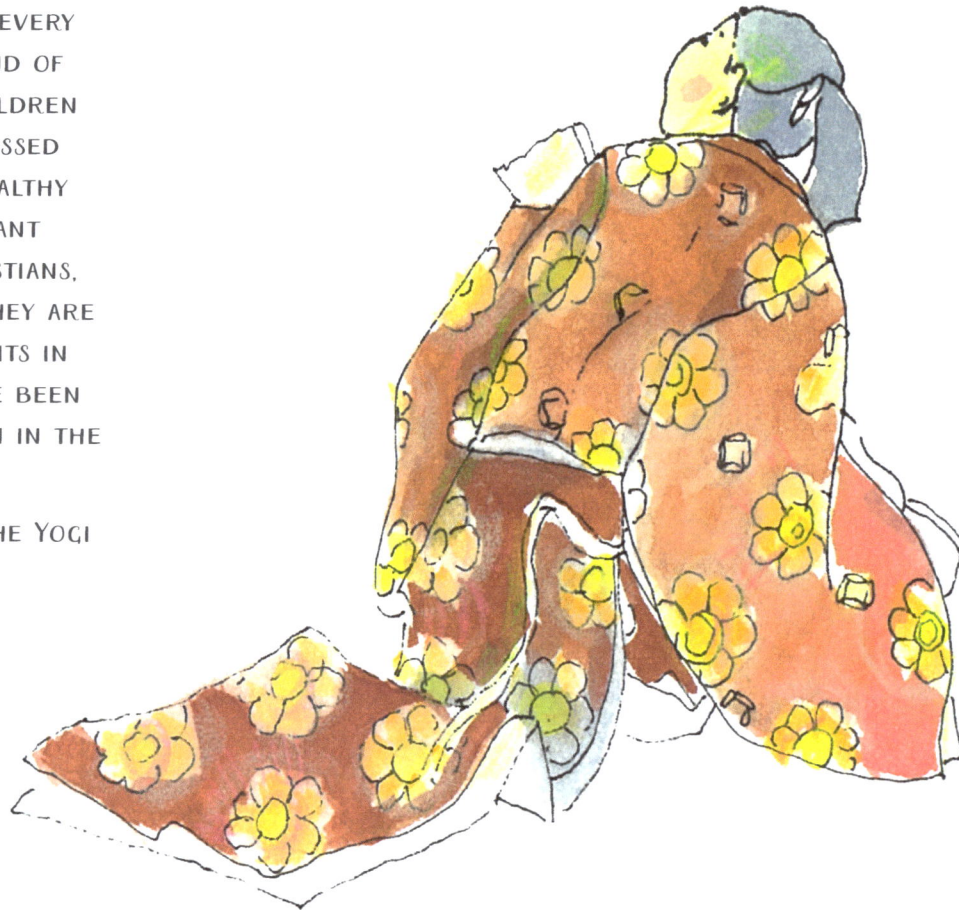

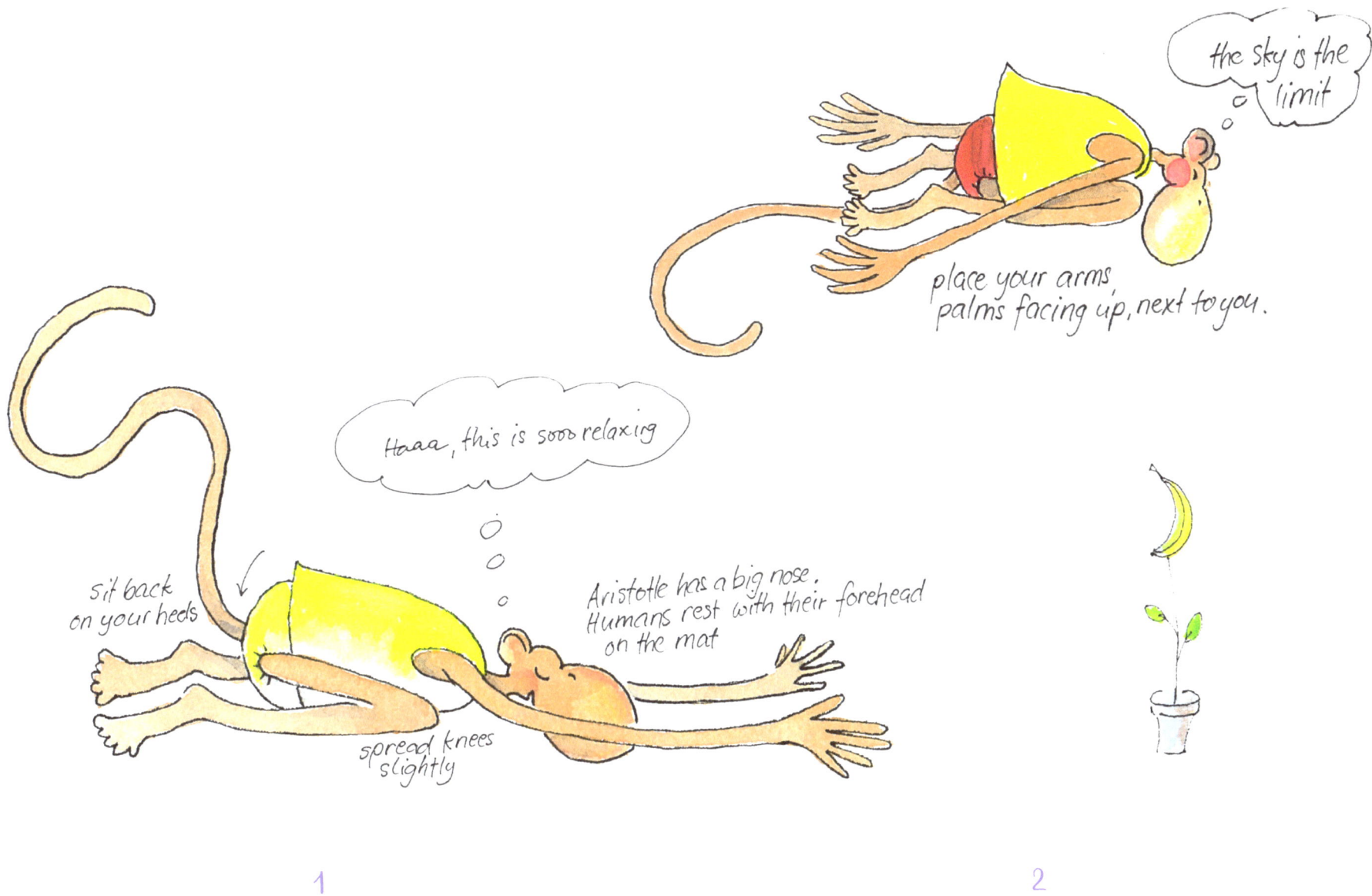

the sky is the limit

place your arms, palms facing up, next to you.

Haaa, this is sooo relaxing

sit back on your heels

Aristotle has a big nose. Humans rest with their forehead on the mat

spread knees slightly

1

Any time you feel the need to rest, come into child's pose. Sit back on your heels and spread your knees slightly apart. Rest on your forehead.

2

Let your chest rest on your thighs. Rest your arms next to the body as in this picture, or extend them in front of you. "Haaaaaaaaaaaa," this is so relaxing.

downward-facing dog

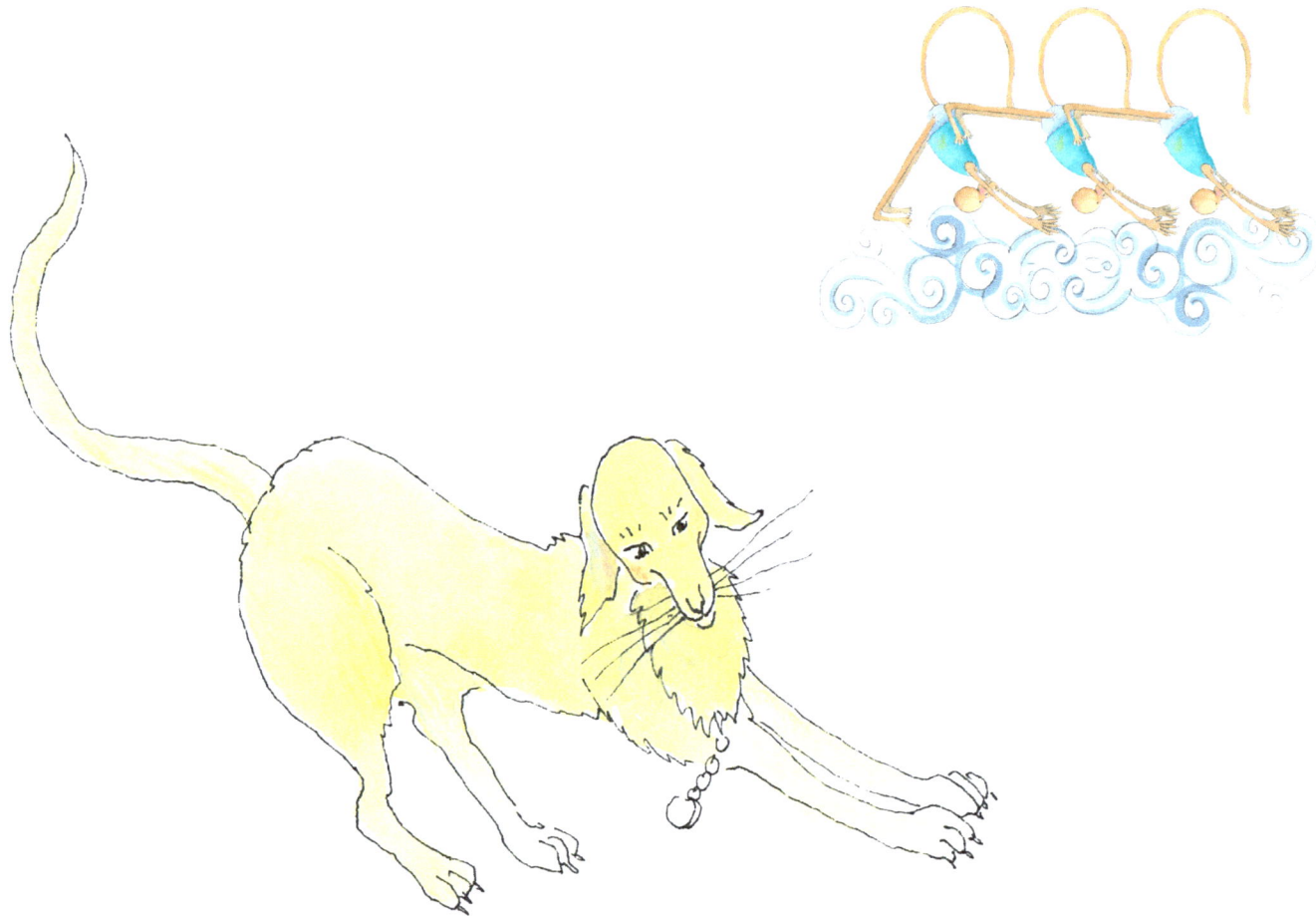

ZEN POINT

Think positively. Who was it that said
you can't teach an old dog new tricks?

MINDFUL FACT

Don't forget to keep loving your dog as he grows
older even though he doesn't look quite as cute. For
centuries, and for good reasons, dogs have been
considered man's best friend.

This pose stretches the entire backside, the arms, shoulders, hips, hamstrings, calves and the back of the heels. It strengthens the arms, hands and the upper body. It's great for the lungs and opens the chest. This is a great warm-up pose and part of the sun salutation.

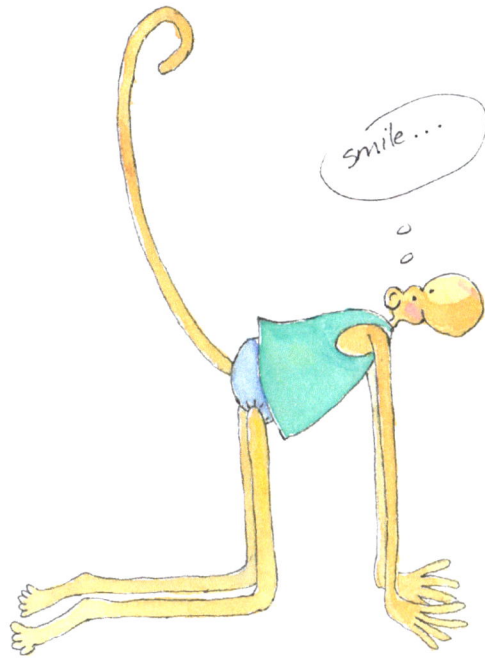

smile . . .

1

Come into cat pose first with your knees hip-width apart.

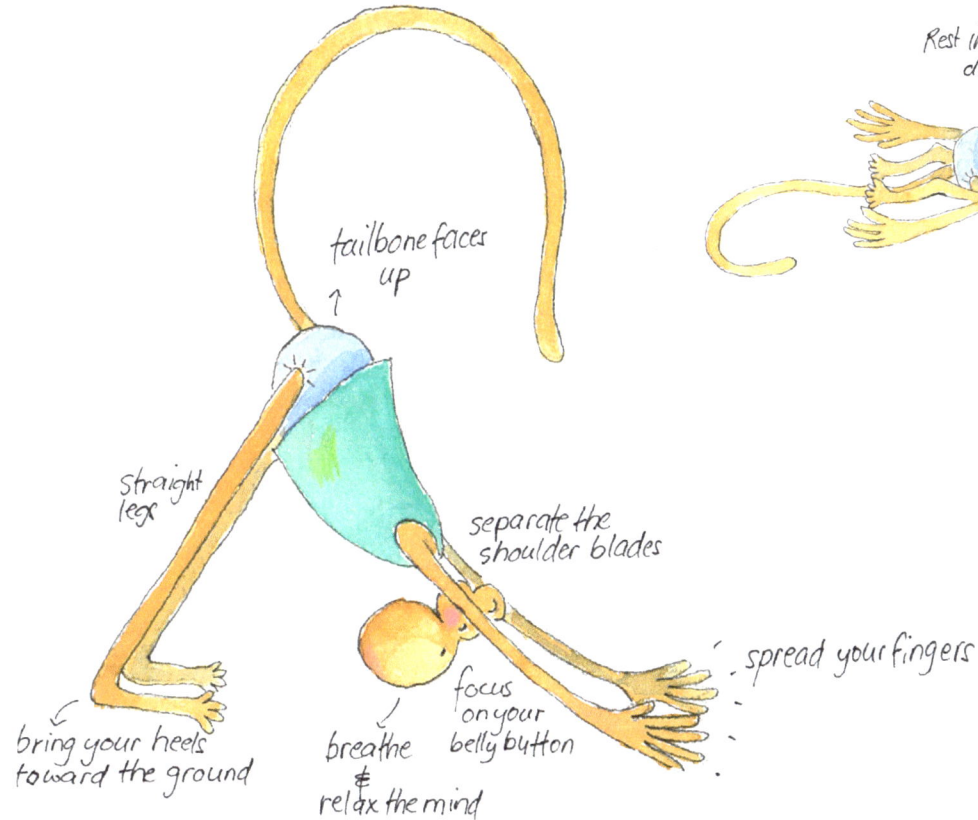

tailbone faces up

straight legs

separate the shoulder blades

spread your fingers

bring your heels toward the ground

breathe & relax the mind

focus on your belly button

2

Now tuck your toes under and lift your bottom up toward the ceiling. At first, it's probably a little difficult to straighten the back of the legs. Focus on lengthening the back and opening your shoulder blades.

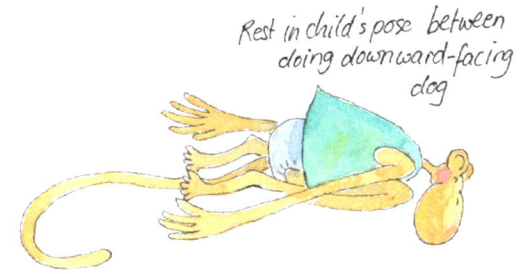

Rest in child's pose between doing downward-facing dog

Gently paddle your feet as you breathe. Never push too hard. Count to 20 or take 5 in and out breaths and then rest. Repeat this pose 3 times.

standing mountain

Standing properly and distributing the weight evenly through your feet keeps your spine elastic and your posture healthy.

MINDFUL FACT

It takes about 3 to 6 weeks to form a good habit. Keep going from there on.

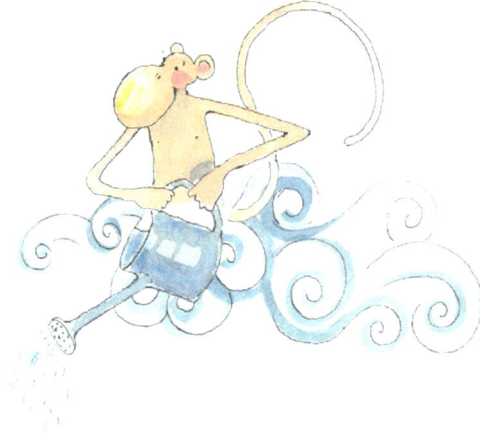

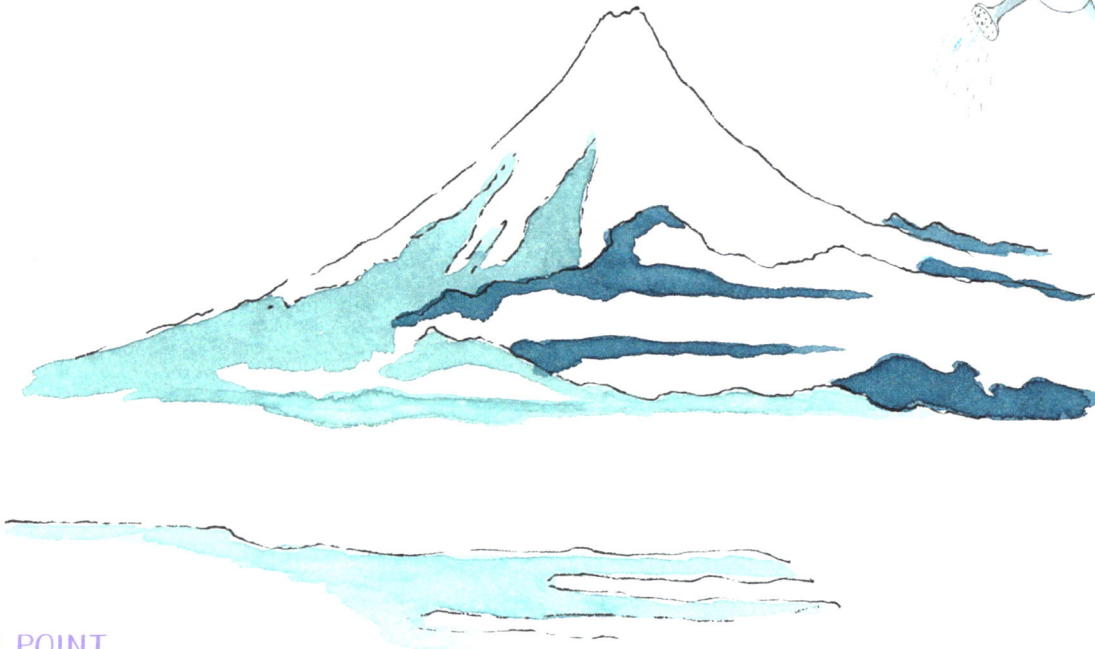

ZEN POINT

A still mind is like a majestic mountain reflecting in a lake.

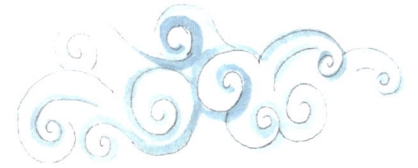

Smile and let any worries
go, go, go....

start to engage
in even breathing
(through the nose)

shoulders are rolled
back

the back is nice & straight

tailbone faces down

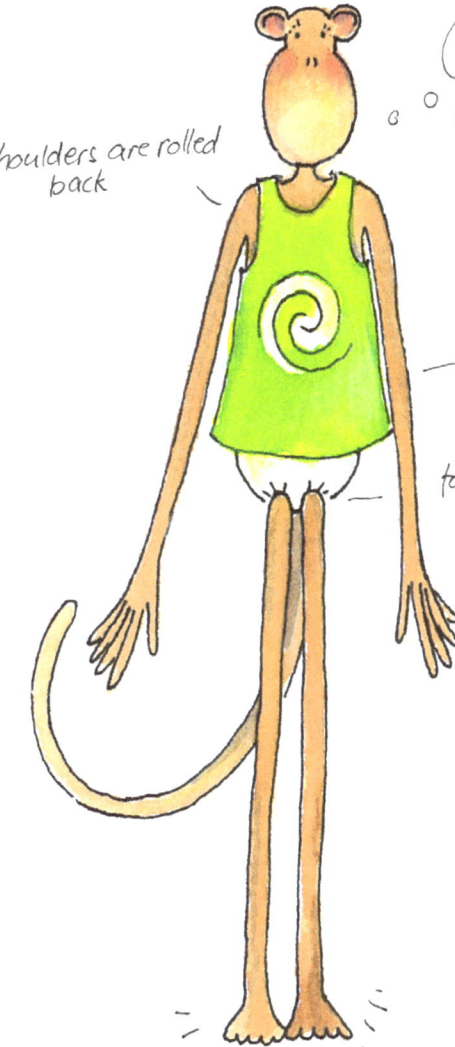

1

Stand straight with your
feet together. Make sure
your heels and toes are flat
on the floor. Balance and
concentration are the key.

2

Place arms, like in the
picture, next to your body.
Many of the poses start off
in standing mountain.

feet are firmly planted into the mat

rising sun salutation

Children should breathe naturally. Generally, as the body stretches we breathe in and as we bend we breathe out. Breath should not be held during any stretch, keep breathing in a stretch.

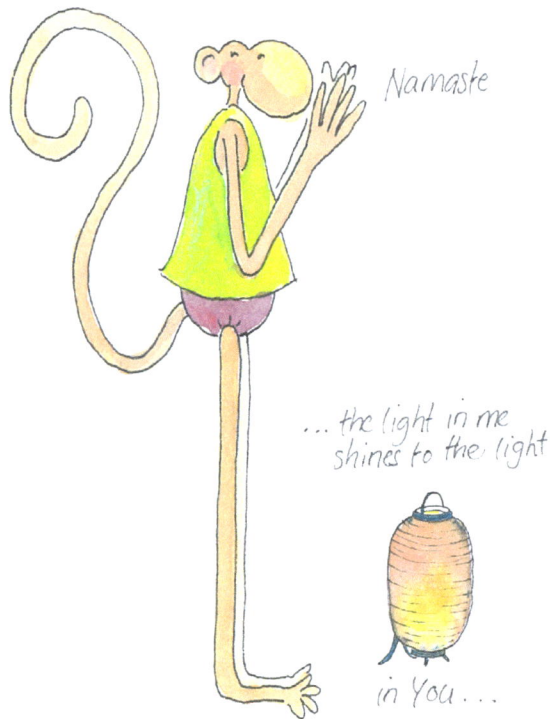

Namaste

... the light in me shines to the light in You ...

reach up to the stars ☆

take a deep breath in... as you stretch

roll your shoulders back

open your ♡

Doing forward bend 3 minutes daily helps positivity...

at first you can bend your knees slightly...

breathe out as you bend forward...

if you can't reach your toes... grab your ankles.

1

Start in standing mountain pose with your feet parallel and your hands to your heart. "Namaste."

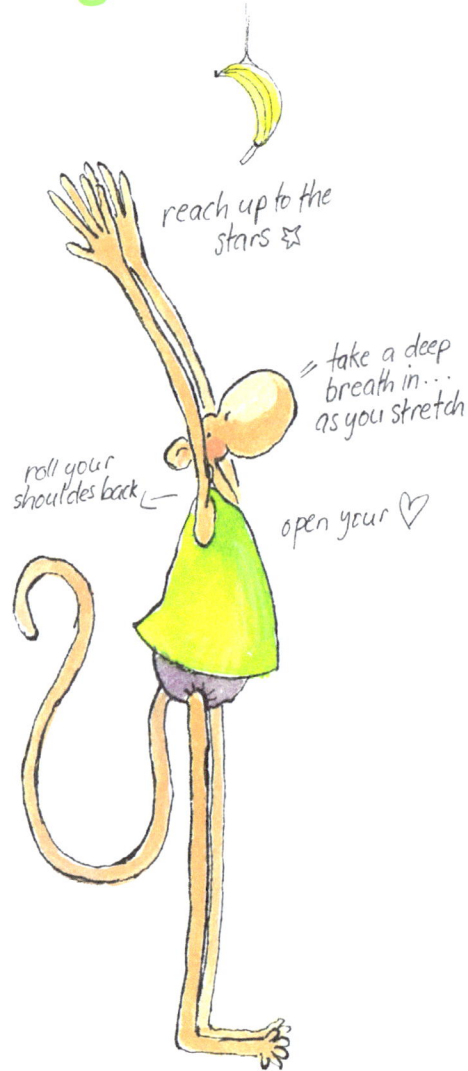

2

Now raise your arms above your head without hunching your shoulders and gently gaze up.

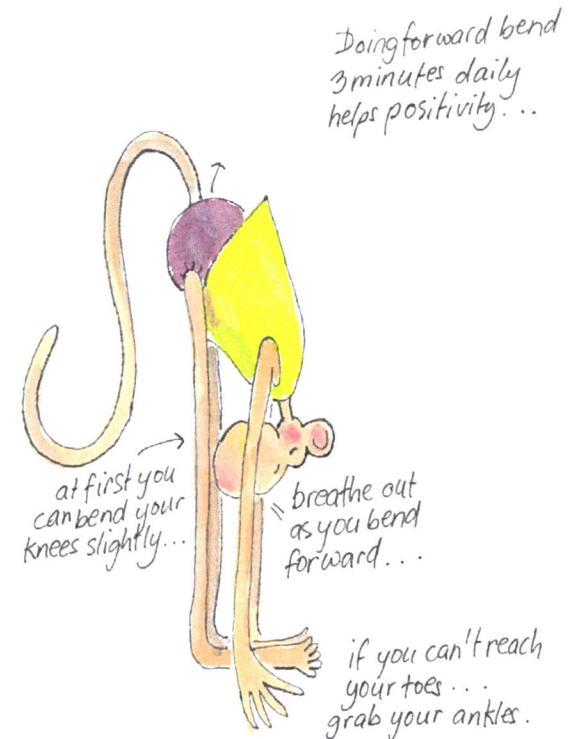

3

Now bend forward from the hips. Keep your knees slightly bent if you feel stiff. This pose is called forward bend.

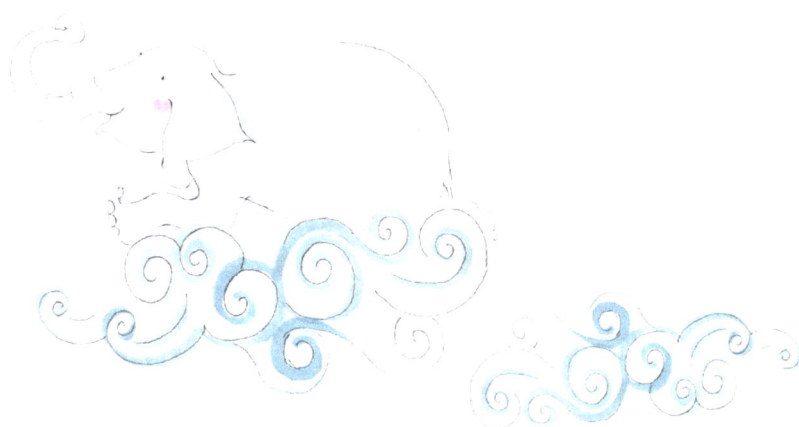

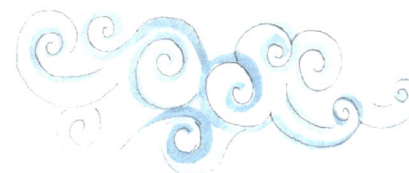

How could we live without
the sun? No trees could
grow and the animals
wouldn't know where to go.

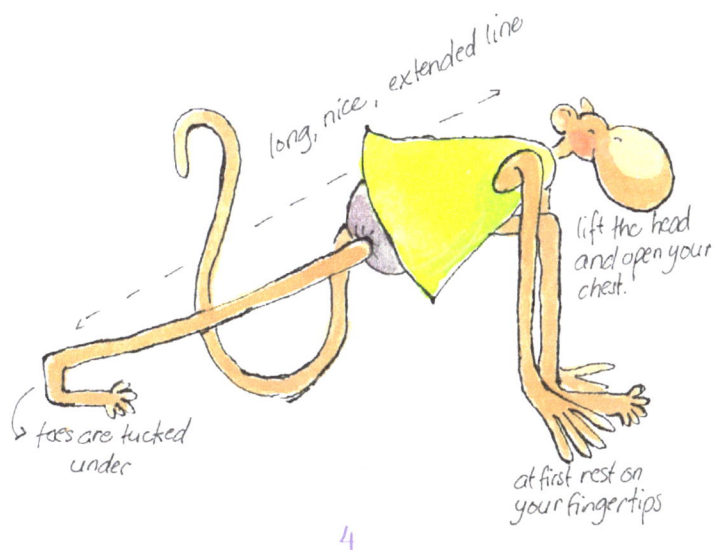

long, nice, extended line

lift the head
and open your
chest.

toes are tucked
under

at first rest on
your fingertips

4

Next, extend your right leg back into
lunge pose with the toes tucked under.
Keep your front foot between the hands.

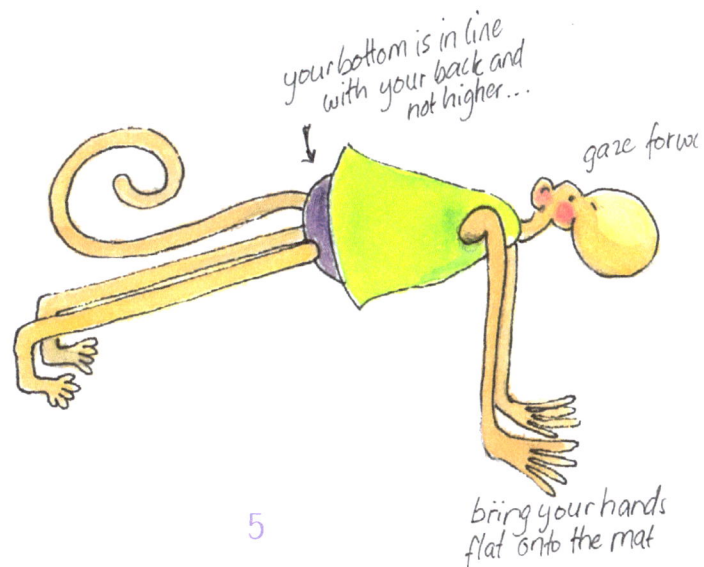

your bottom is in line
with your back and
not higher...

gaze forwa

bring your hands
flat onto the mat

5

Now bring both feet back into
plank pose. Keep your arms
and belly strong.

23

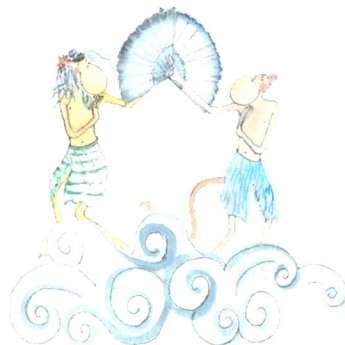

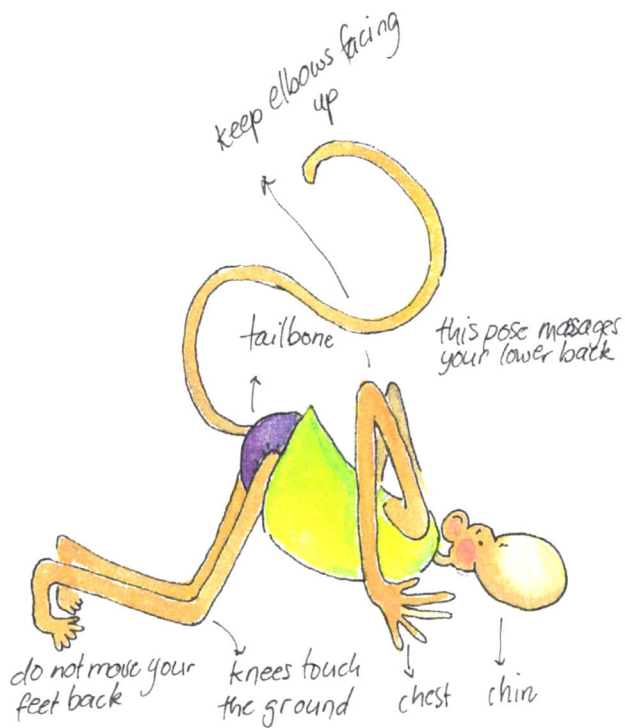

keep elbows facing up

tailbone

this pose massages your lower back

do not move your feet back

knees touch the ground

chest

chin

Aristotle's tail tingles. He loves cobra pose!

gaze up

elbows stay in and face up

open and lift the ♡

toes are now pointing away from the body

hands are pushed into the mat

6

7

Now breathe out, bringing your knees and then the chest and chin to the floor without moving your hands or feet.

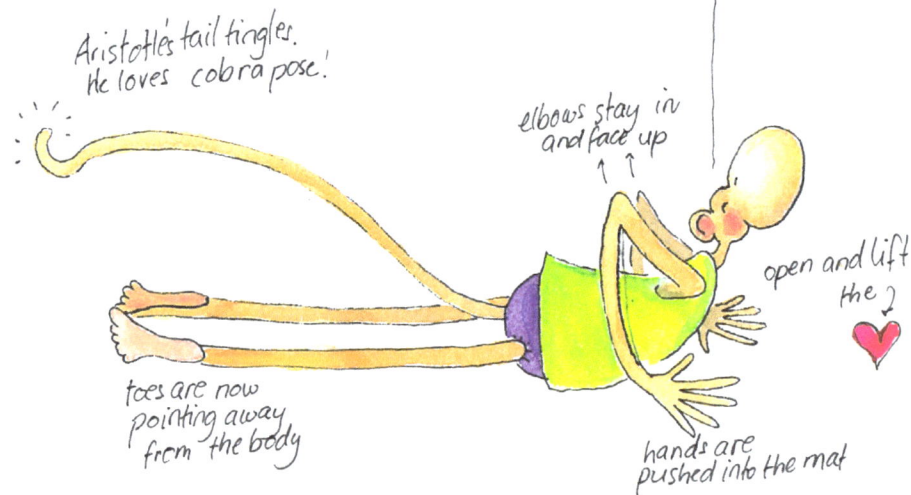

Now lift your chest up between your hands and stretch into cobra pose. Keep shoulders rolled back.

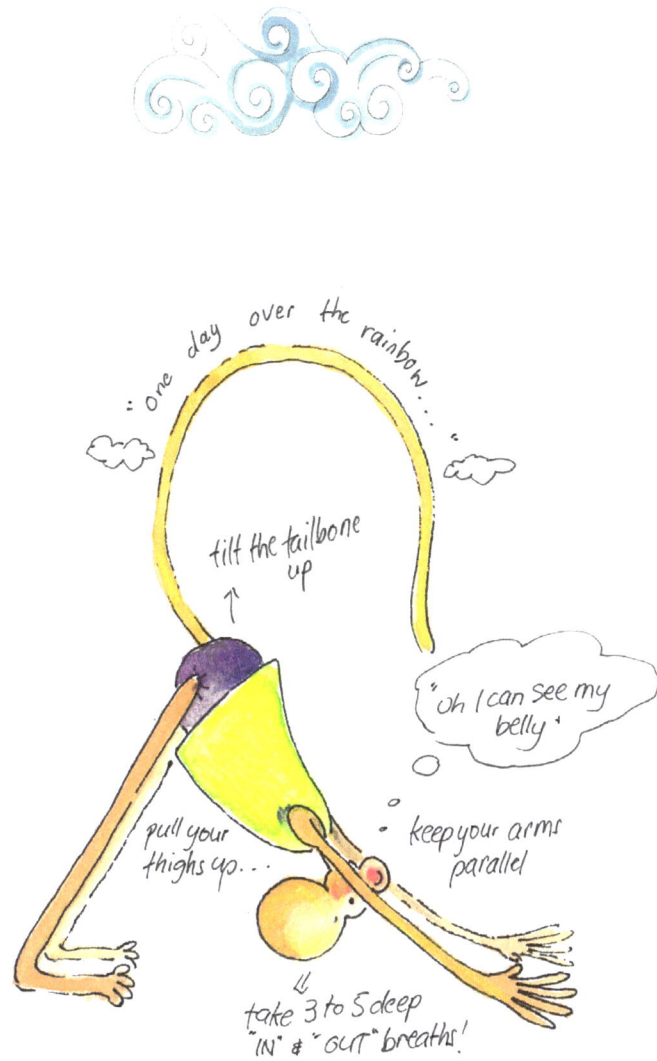

One day over the rainbow...

tilt the tailbone up ↑

"oh I can see my belly"

pull your thighs up...

keep your arms parallel

take 3 to 5 deep "IN" & "OUT" breaths!

8

Next, tuck your toes under and lift your bottom up into downward-facing dog. Keep your head down and count to 10 as you breathe or take 3 to 5 in and out breaths.

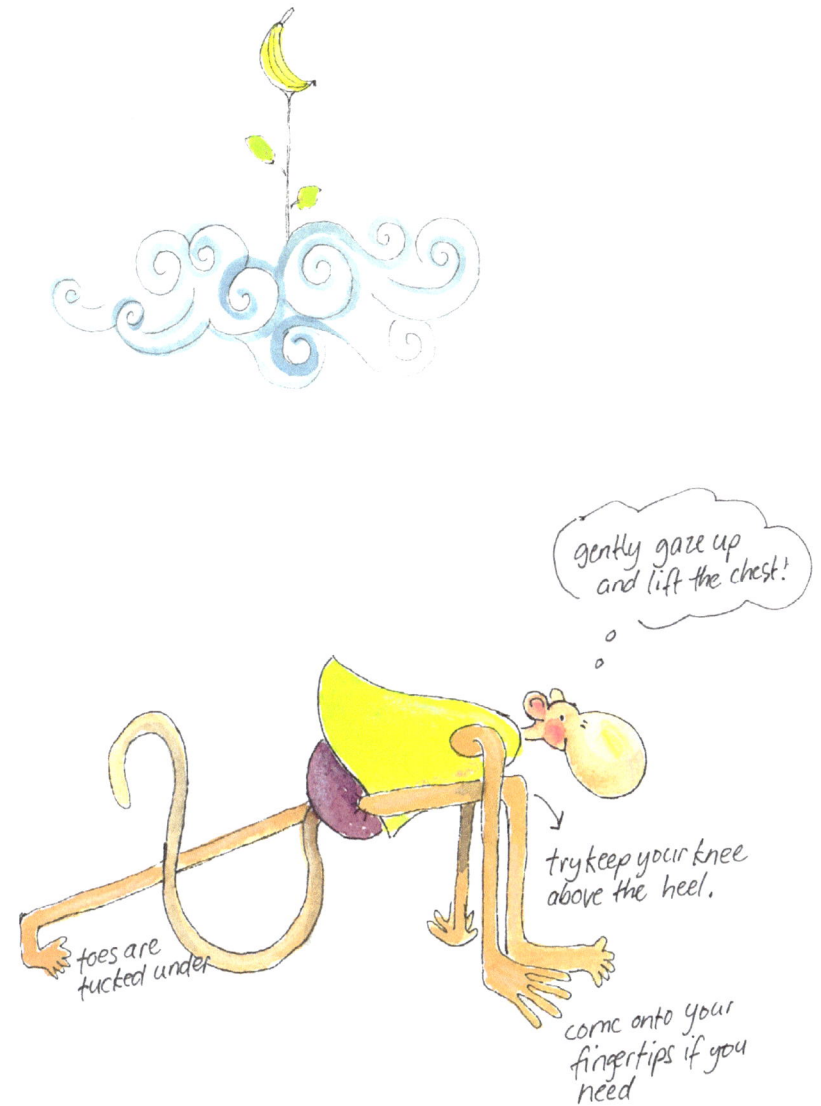

gently gaze up and lift the chest!

try keep your knee above the heel.

toes are tucked under

come onto your fingertips if you need

9

Now step the right leg between your hands into lunge pose. Rest on your fingertips for an easier stretch. Smile.

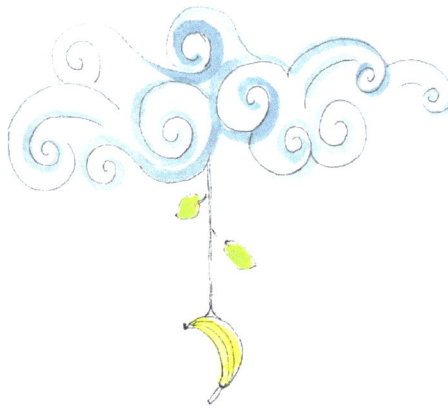

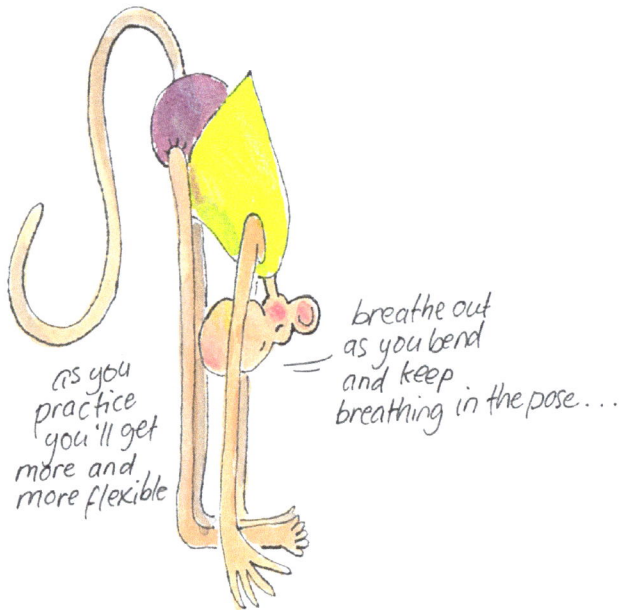

breathe in
as you reach up . . .

♡ listen to the
music in your
soul . . .

as you
practice
you'll get
more and
more flexible

breathe out
as you bend
and keep
breathing in the pose . . .

10

11

Now step both legs between your hands and
bend into forward bend once more. You should
feel a bit more flexible this time around.

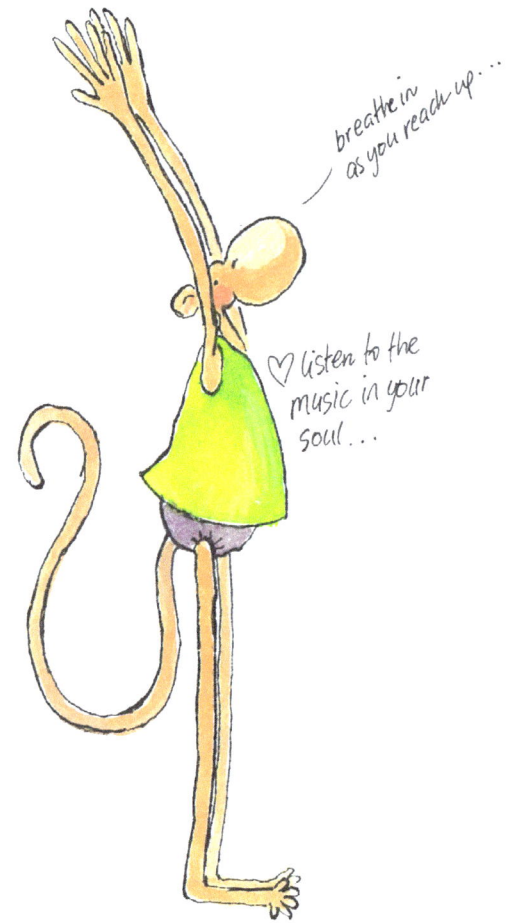

Take a deep breath and lift your
arms the same way as before.

"HERE COMES THE SUN LITTLE DARLING"...

"Namaste"

keep the light in your heart shining...

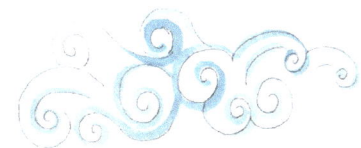

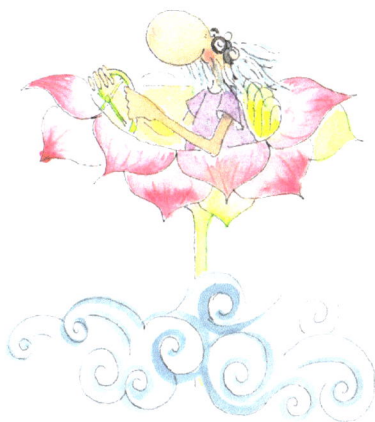

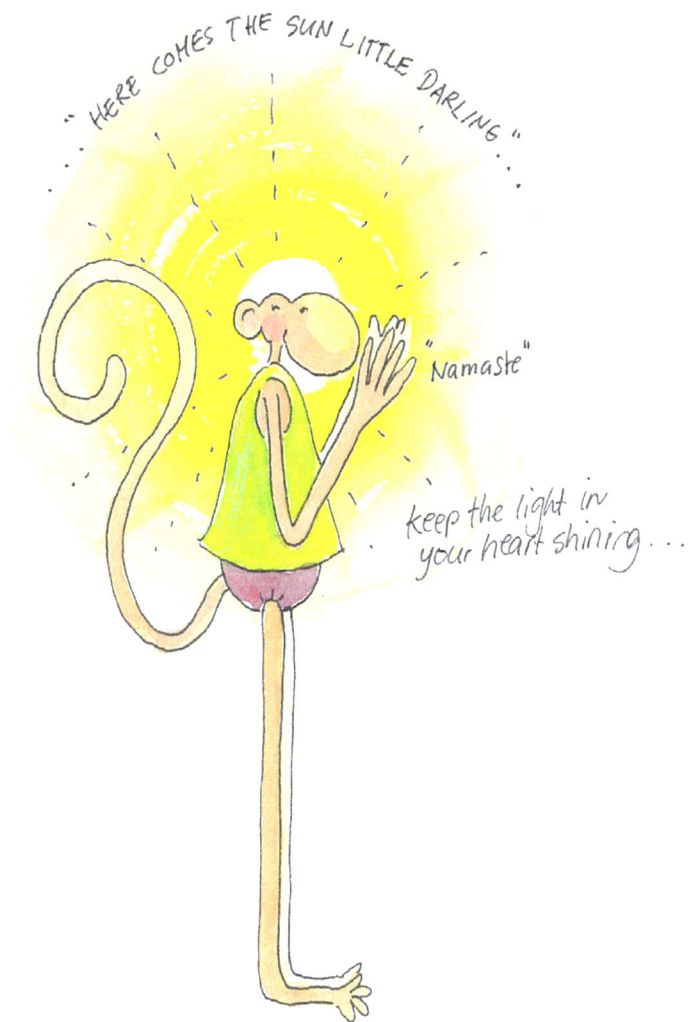

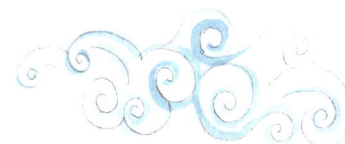

Do the rising sun salutation 3 to 6 times. It will make you more flexible and really heat the fire in your belly.

12

Relax and come into standing mountain pose bringing your hands to your heart. "Namaste."

simple standing flow sequence—
bringing in the standing poses

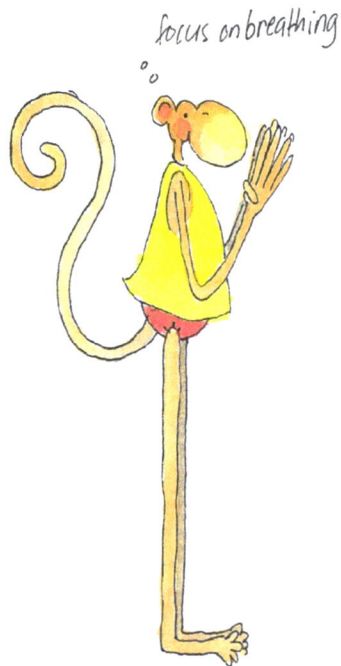

focus on breathing

arms parallel to the mat

palms face down

turn both feet as in the picture

lift your arms shoulder-width apart or bring your palms together...

1

Start in standing mountain pose with hands to your heart. "Namaste."

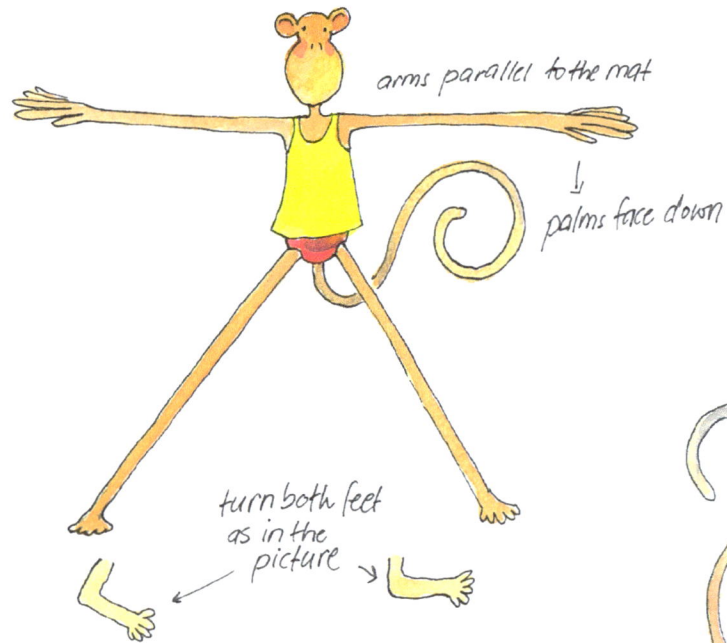

2

Jump your feet apart so you are standing sideways on the mat. Don't forget to breathe.

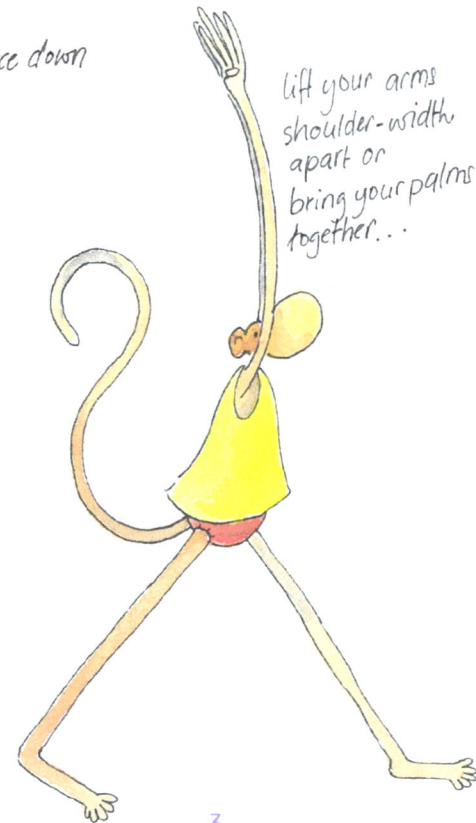

3

Now turn your left foot to the front and your back foot in the same direction at a comfy angle. Square hips forward. Now take a deep breath and sweep your arms up palms facing each other.

4

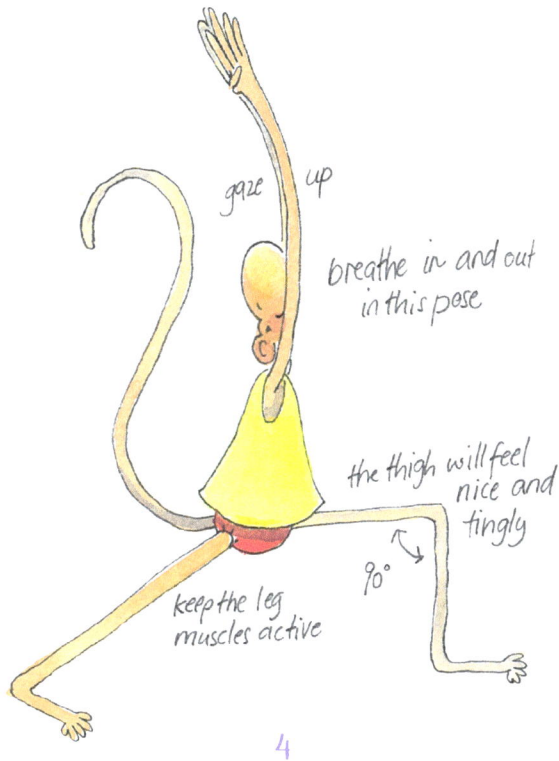

Bend your front knee at a 90-degree angle making sure your knee stays above the heel. Keep the back leg straight. Lift the gaze toward your fingertips. Take 3 to 5 in and out breaths, or count to 10 as you breathe. Don't forget to smile.

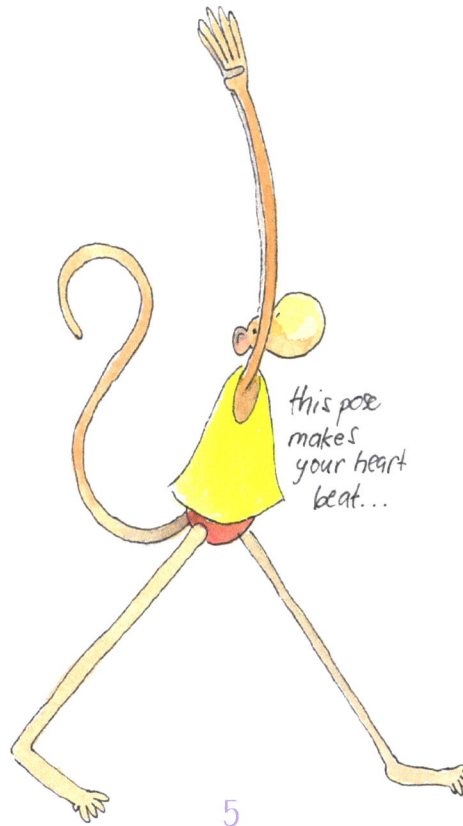

5

Now straighten the front leg.

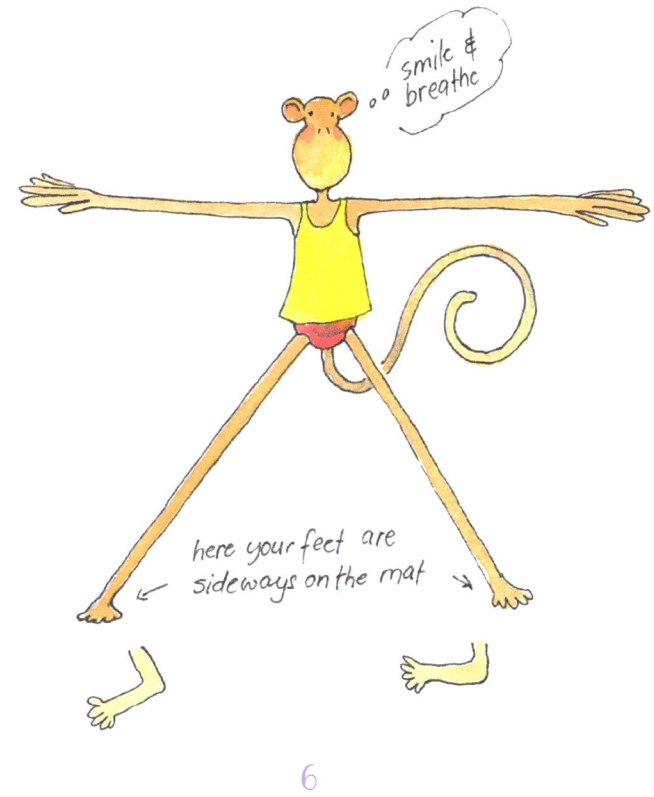

6

Come back to the centre position with your arms parallel to the mat. Turn your feet in the opposite direction . . .

Study the various warrior poses and bring them into this simple flowing sequence.

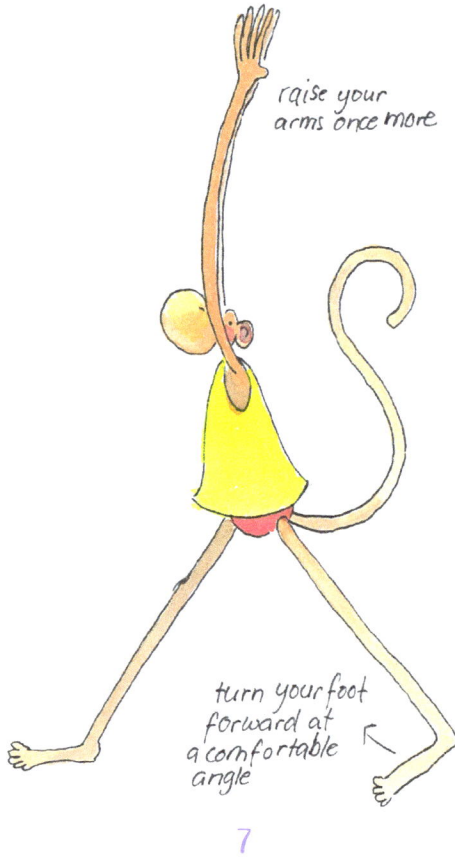

This pose is called Warrior I

raise your arms once more

The knee comes above the heel..

90°
keep both legs active!

8

Bend your other front leg forming a 90-degree angle as you raise your arms above the head. Gaze toward your finger tips and don't forget to breathe as you count to 10.

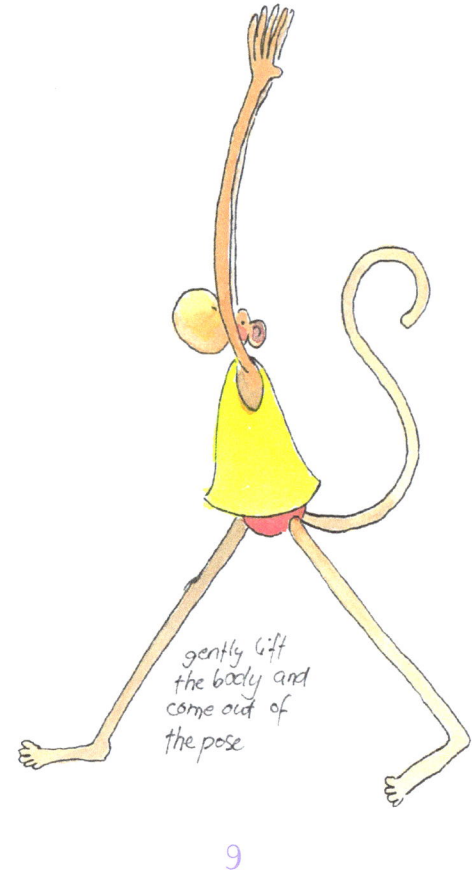

turn your foot forward at a comfortable angle

gently lift the body and come out of the pose

7

9

At this point rotate your heels in the opposite direction.

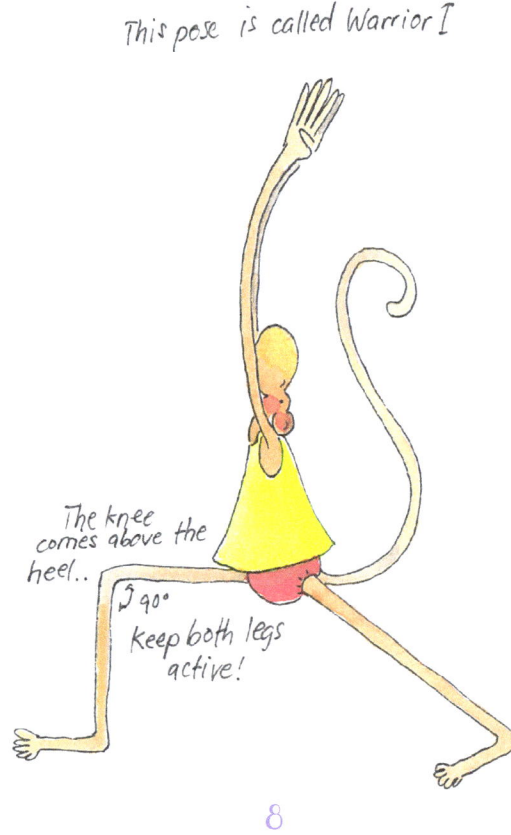

Now straighten the front leg once more.

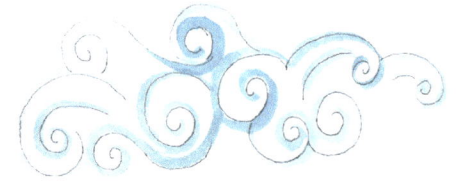

imagine!
an invisible string
pulling   you gently
up

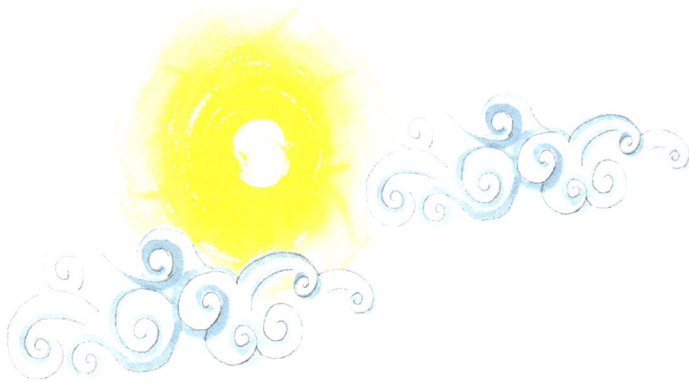

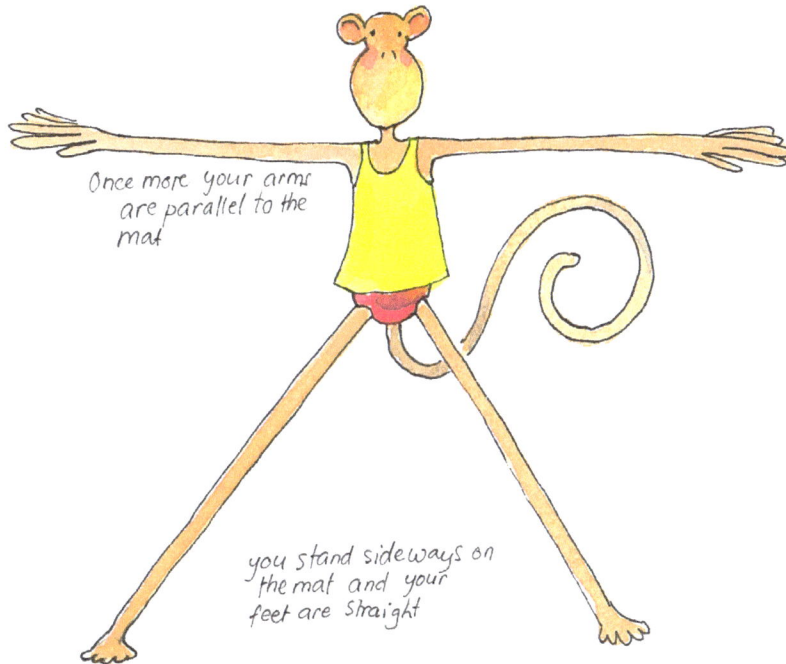

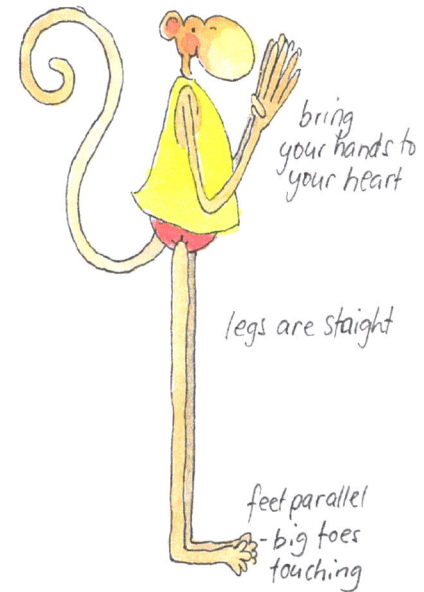

Once more your arms
are parallel to the
mat

bring
your hands to
your heart

legs are straight

you stand sideways on
the mat and your
feet are straight

feet parallel
-big toes
touching

10

11

Turn your feet so you are standing facing
the long side of the mat, holding your
arms back out to the side . . .

. . . and last but not least, jump
your feet together towards the front
of the mat. Well done.

triangle pose

This pose shapes your legs nicely and helps a tired back and neck. Monkeys living in the wilderness don't usually suffer from these problems.

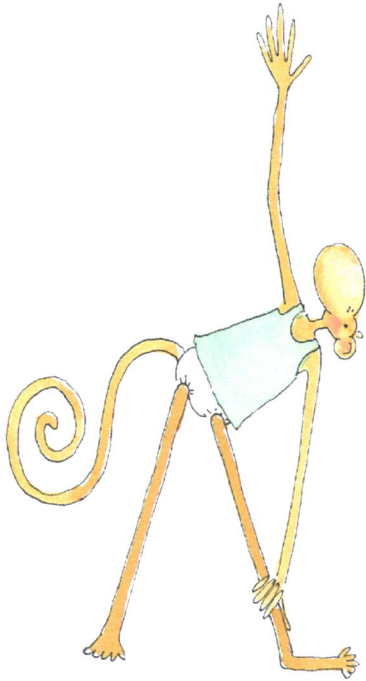

MINDFUL FACT

A little effort is needed to keep going. Come on, you can do it.

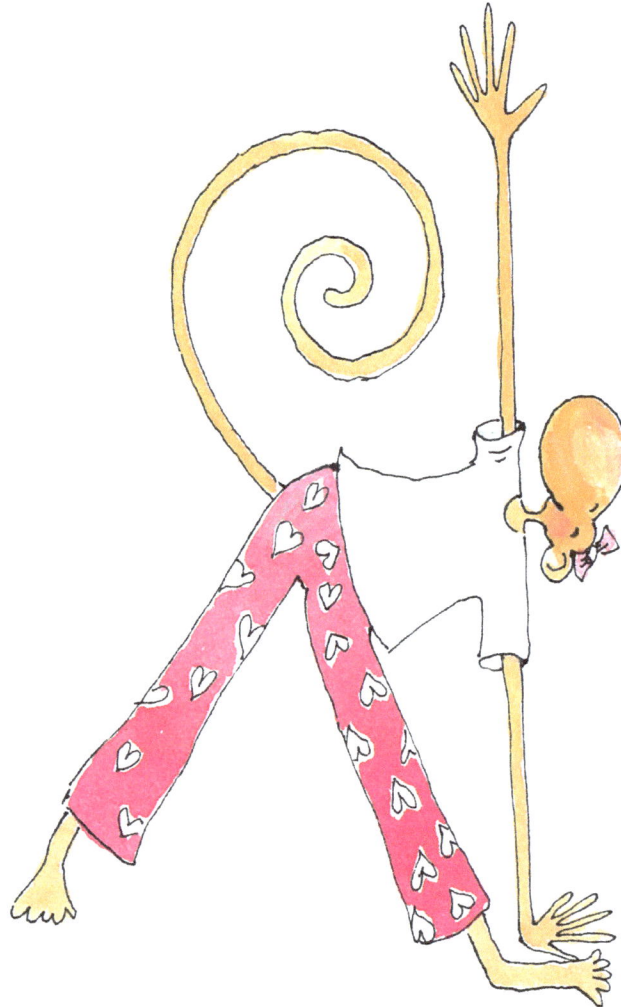

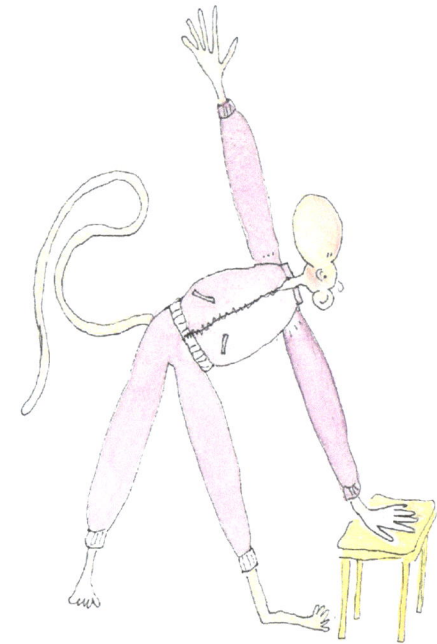

ZEN POINT

Don't worry if you can't reach down to the floor in this pose, rest the hand on your leg or a chair. We're all different so listen to your body and heart.

Now it's getting exciting and rather lively. Remember monkeys have long arms so it is easy for them to reach the floor.

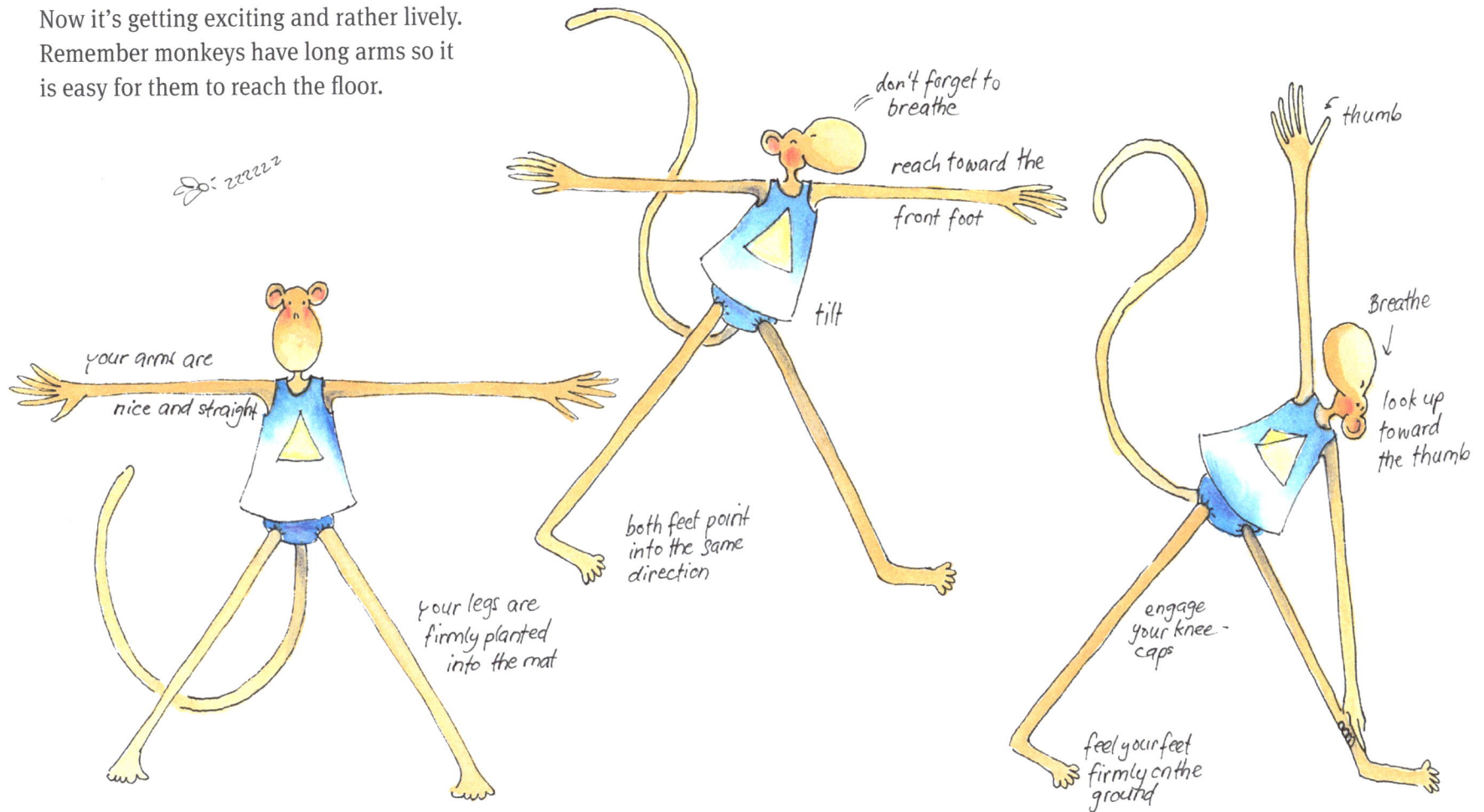

zzzzzz

your arms are nice and straight

your legs are firmly planted into the mat

don't forget to breathe

reach toward the front foot

tilt

both feet point into the same direction

thumb

Breathe

look up toward the thumb

engage your knee caps

feel your feet firmly on the ground

1

Start in standing mountain pose with your hands in Namaste. Now jump your feet apart so you stand sideways on the mat. Lift your arms parallel and spread your fingers.

2

Turn both feet forward as in the picture, and then reach as far as you can toward the direction of your front foot.

3

Now tilt sideways and see if you can reach your ankle. Only reach as far as is comfortable and gaze up. Count to 10. Stand up, rotate the heels and do the same on the other side.

extended side-angle pose

MINDFUL FACT

Try being enthusiastic about what you do. Sometimes it feels like you're faking it. But do it anyway; it's like yawning, it's infectious.

Builds strong ankles, knees and thighs and keeps your waist nice and trim. It also helps the digestion.

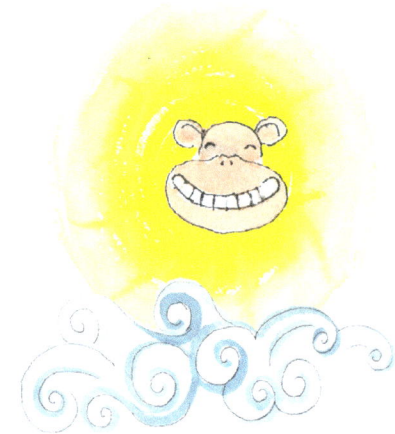

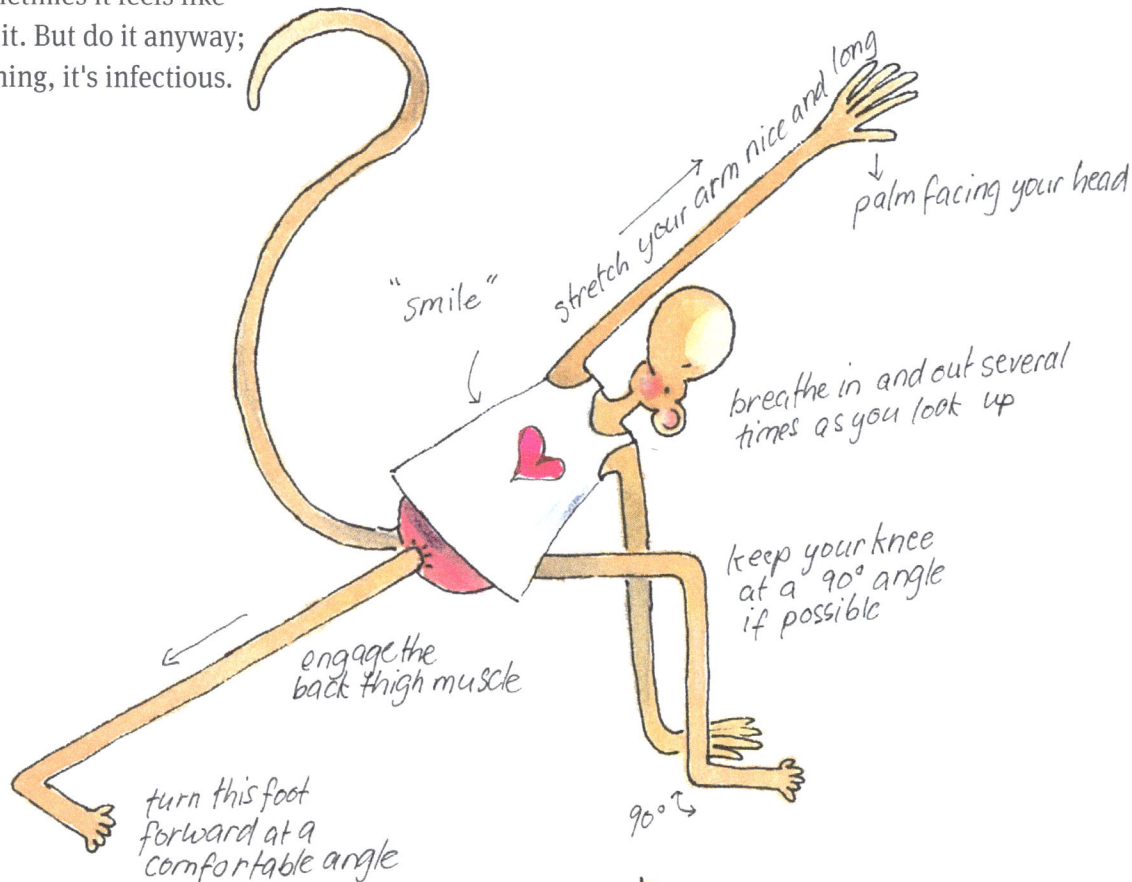

"smile"

stretch your arm nice and long

palm facing your head

breathe in and out several times as you look up

keep your knee at a 90° angle if possible

engage the back thigh muscle

turn this foot forward at a comfortable angle

90°

1

Start in standing mountain pose and jump your feet apart so you stand sideways on the mat.

Bend your front knee at a 90-degree angle. Both feet are turned toward the front of the mat and flat on the floor.

2

Place the left hand on the outside of the bent front leg and reach past your head with the right arm. Look up toward the upper palm and breathe.

Now come out of the pose and repeat on the other side.

twisted side-angle pose

This pose works wonders on your spinal column and abdominal organs. It helps if you suffer from constipation!

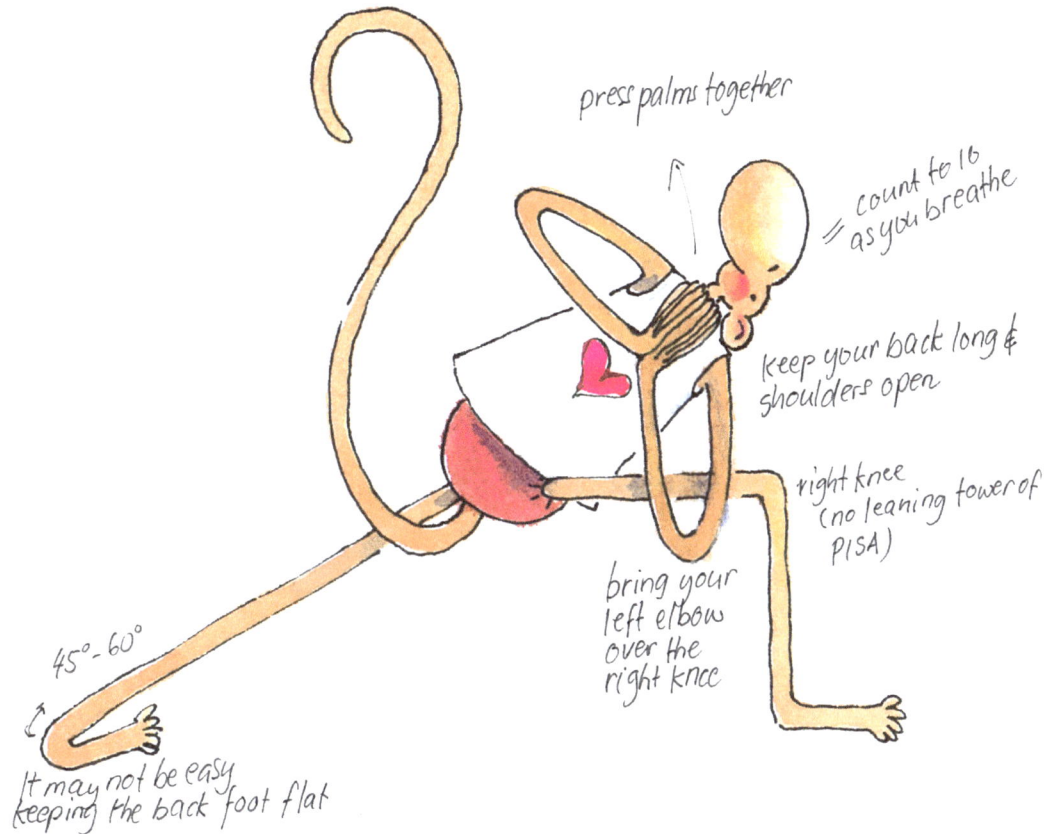

press palms together

count to 16 as you breathe

keep your back long & shoulders open

right knee (no leaning tower of PISA)

bring your left elbow over the right knee

45° - 60°

It may not be easy keeping the back foot flat

1

Start in standing mountain pose with your hands in Namaste. Now jump your legs apart so you are standing sideways on the mat. Turn your hips forward and bend your right knee at a 90-degree angle. Now bring your left elbow over the outer part of the right thigh.

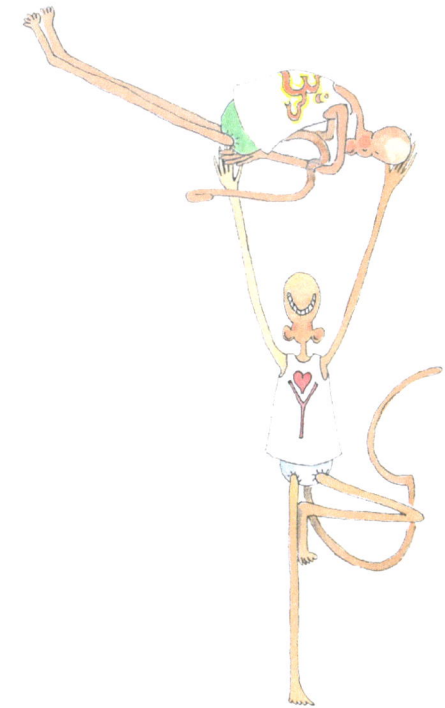

2

Press your palms together and gaze up. Breathe naturally as you count to 10. Smile and repeat the pose on the other side.

warrior I

Warrior I strengthens the legs, shoulders and arms. It gives
you stamina and makes the hips and back more flexible.

It's the beginning of a back-bend pose.

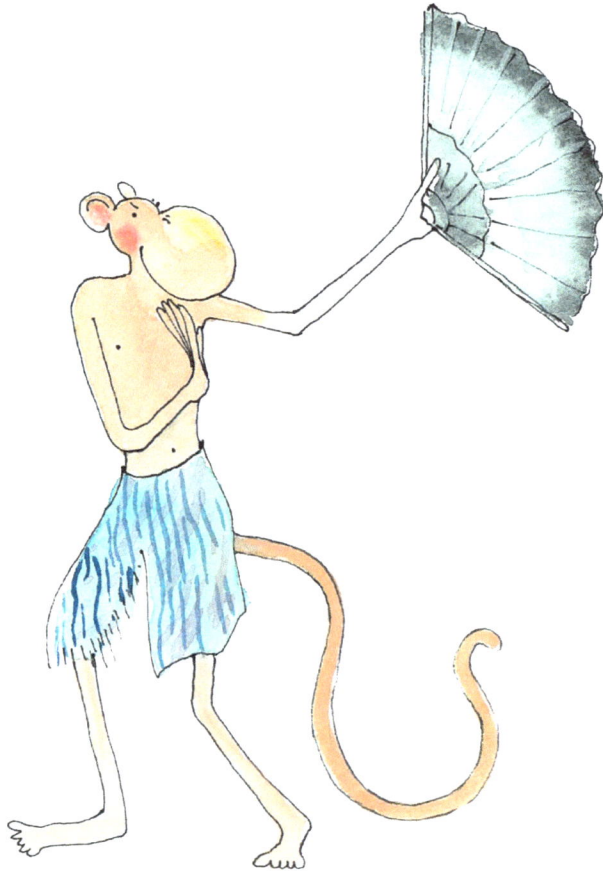

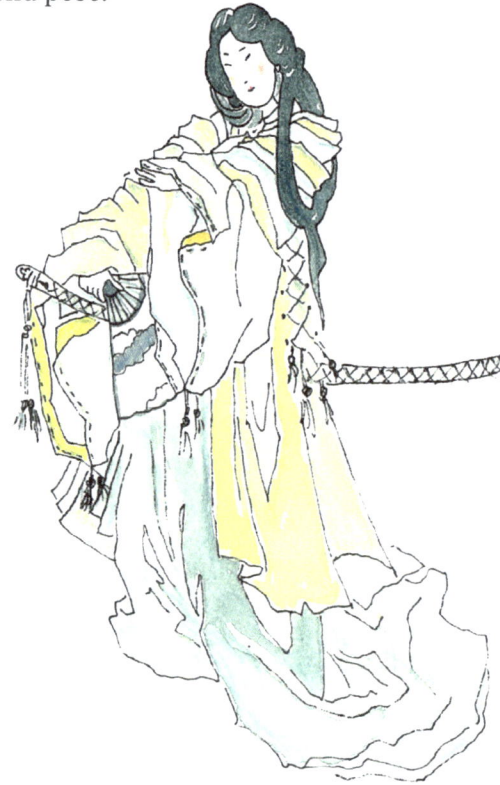

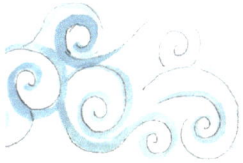

This is the pose from the standing flow sequence.

1

Start in standing mountain and follow the standing flow sequence. Now let's look at the pose in more detail. The back foot is turned forward at a comfortable angle. Hips are facing forward and the front knee is bent at an angle. It shouldn't tilt to either side like the leaning tower of Pisa.

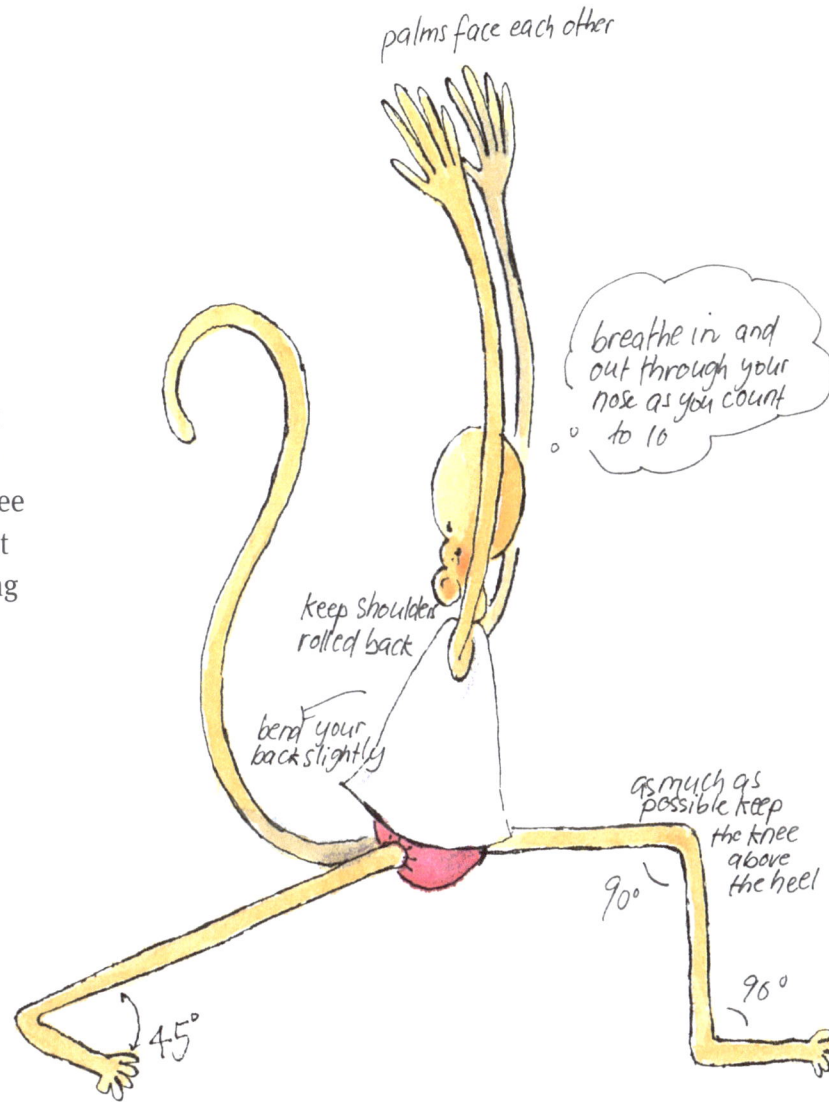

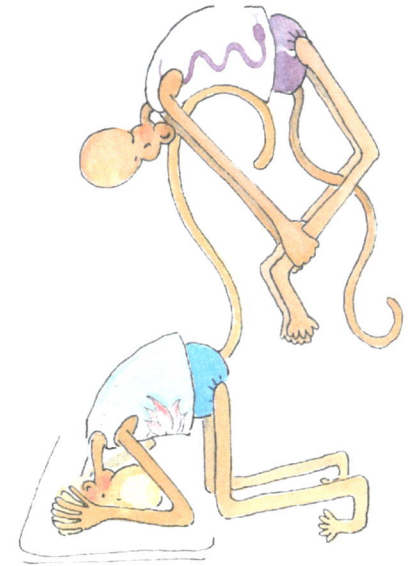

palms face each other

breathe in and out through your nose as you count to 10

keep shoulder rolled back

bend your back slightly

as much as possible keep the knee above the heel

90°

90°

45°

2

Sweep your arms out and up toward the ceiling. You can bring your palms together or keep them shoulder-width apart. Shoulders are rolled back. Gaze up towards your fingertips. Count to 10 or take 3 to 5 deep breaths. Stand strong like a hero and don't forget to smile. Now repeat the pose on the other side.

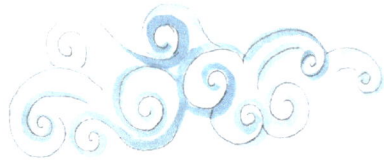

warrior II

This pose increases stamina and makes the legs and heart stronger. It also helps concentration and staying grounded.

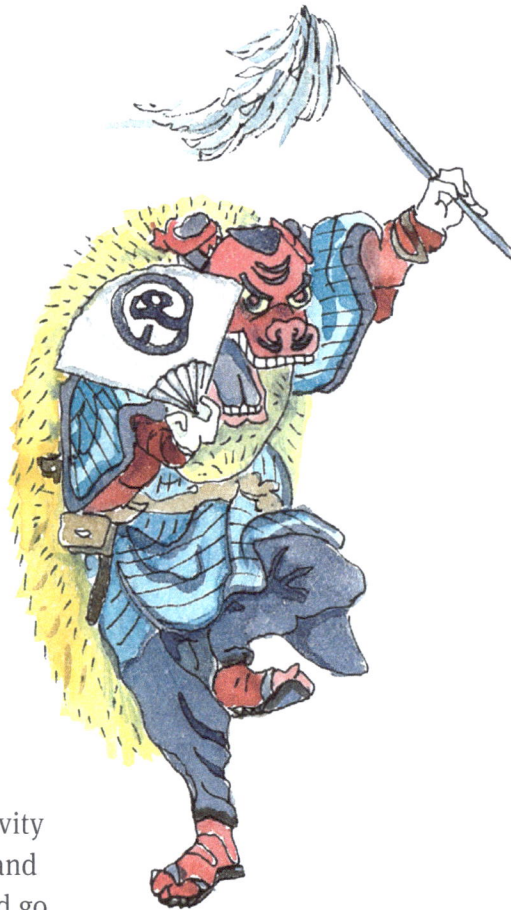

ZEN POINT

Try to perform each activity with your whole heart and if you really feel troubled go find someone who cares to listen wholeheartedly.

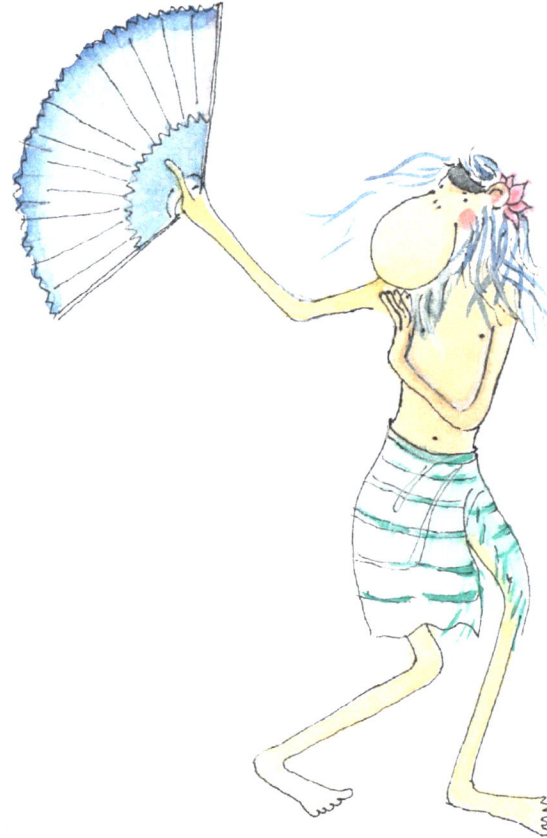

MINDFUL FACT

There are no short cuts in getting a job well done; but it's a lot easier if you're around family and friends who care.

You can come into this pose through the standing flow sequence.

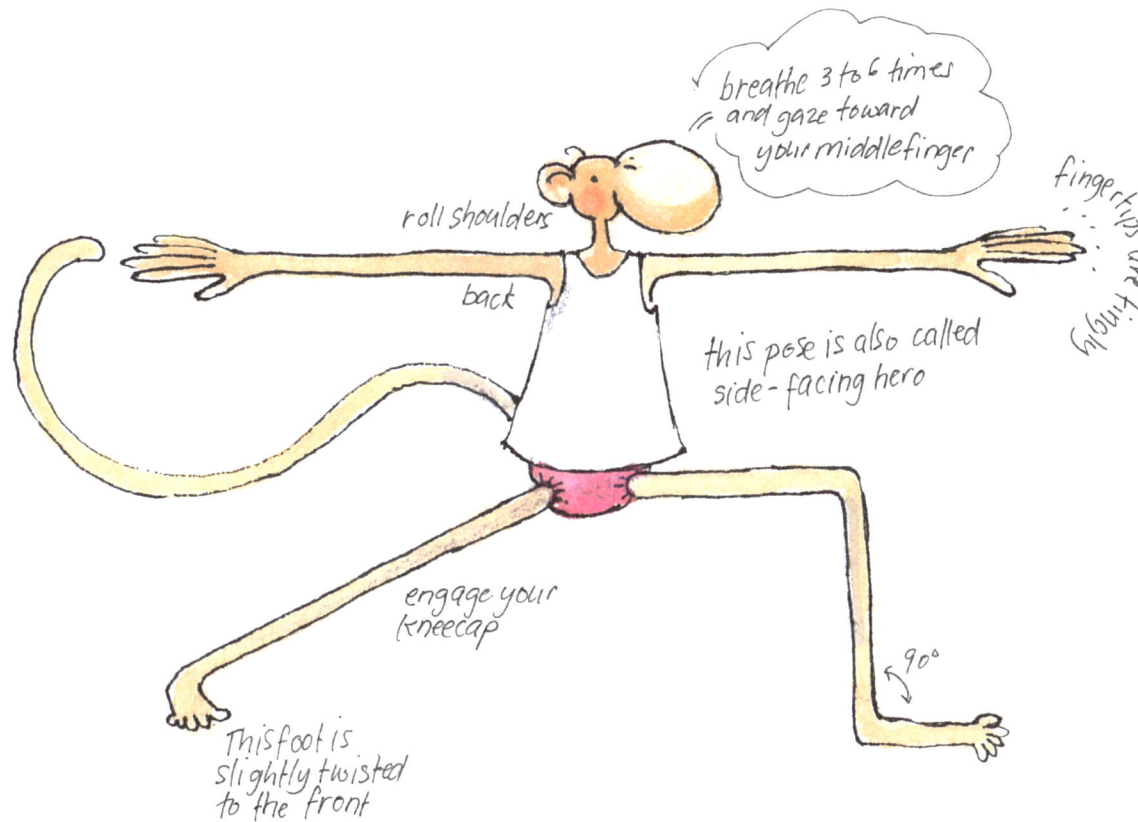

breathe 3 to 6 times and gaze toward your middlefinger

roll shoulders

back

this pose is also called side-facing hero

fingertips are tingly

engage your kneecap

90°

This foot is slightly twisted to the front

1

2

Start in standing mountain pose and jump your feet apart so you are standing sideways on the mat. In warrior II the hips face to the side. As you can see in the picture your back leg is straight and the foot is tilted forward at a comfortable angle. Your arms are lifted parallel to the mat and shoulders are relaxed.

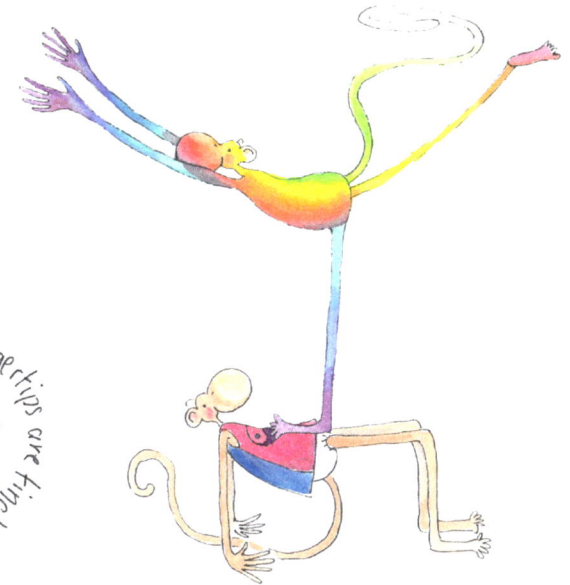

Focus on the middle finger of your front hand. For those of you whose monkey mind is still busy, focus on breathing and smile. Take 3 to 5 deep breaths. Don't forget to repeat the pose facing the other way.

crane pose

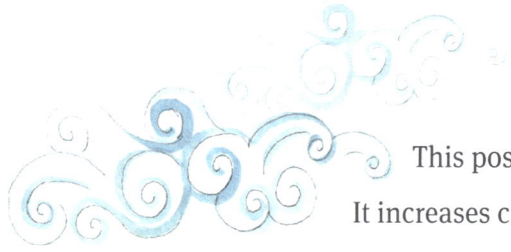

This pose develops the ankles and is great for loosening stiff shoulders.

It increases circulation in the calf muscles and helps unmuddle a muddled mind.

ZEN POINT

Give yourself a chance to see the world through another culture's eyes and be creative about life rather than judge that which is different. Sure, some things are weird, but that's OK too, isn't it? There are weird fish in the ocean and strange insects in the jungle. They too have the right to live just as much as you and me.

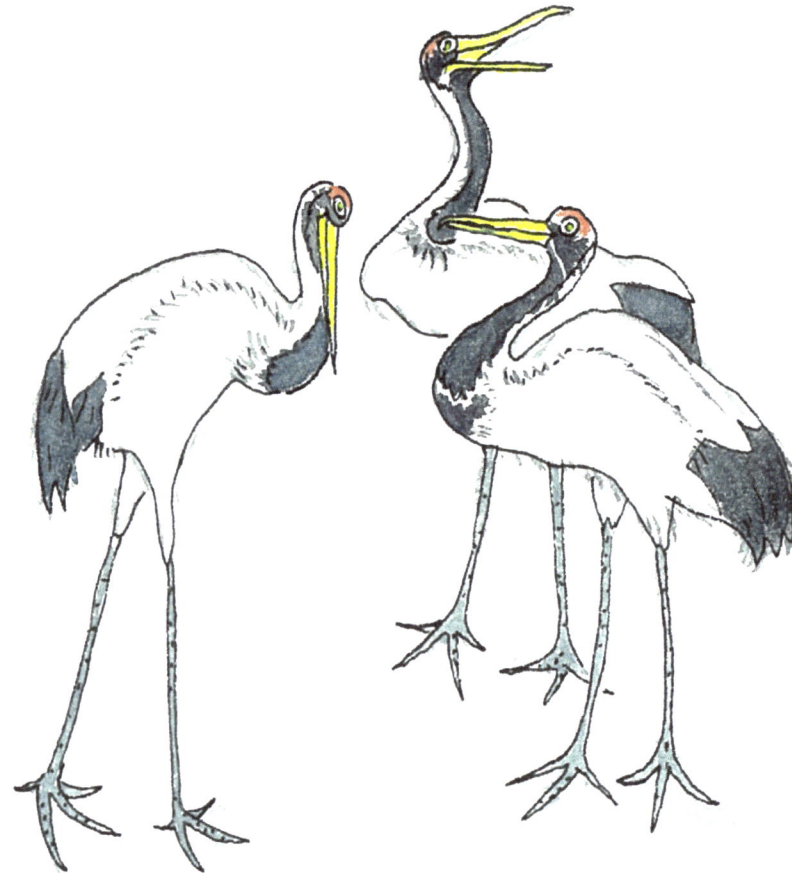

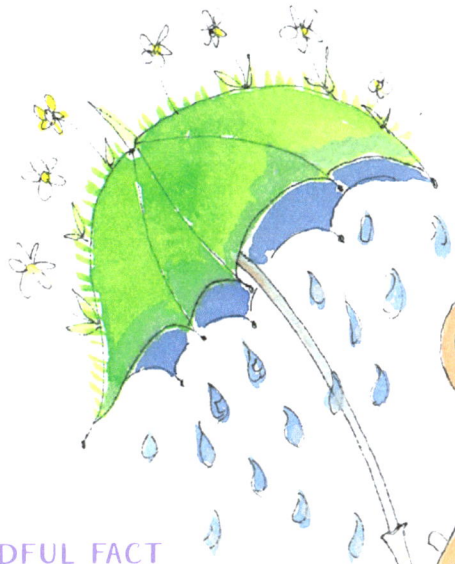

Too many people never try something
they're not familiar with because
they're either too afraid to fail or
maybe even more afraid that they're
actually going to like it.

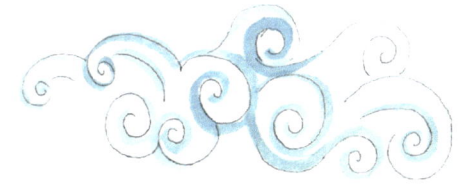

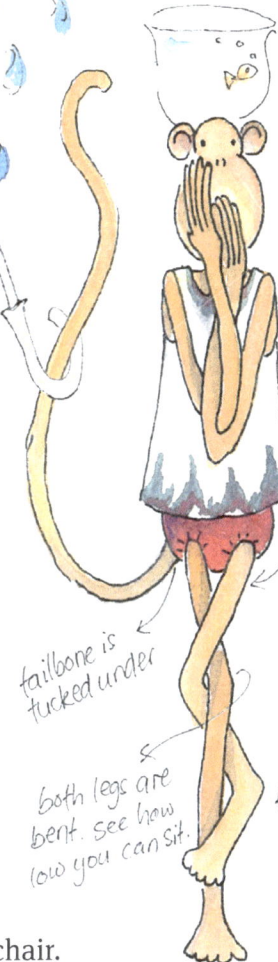

lift the elbows a bit higher

bring your left leg over your right one.

tailbone is tucked under

both legs are bent. see how low you can sit.

the left foot is curled around the right calf.

1

Start by pretending you're sitting down in a chair.
Cross your left leg over your right leg and see if
you can twist further by bringing the right foot
around the left calf. This takes patience and time.
Bend your arms at the elbow and bring the left
arm under the right elbow.

2

Don't change the direction of the hands. See if you can
grab the right thumb with the left hand. Lift your elbows
up to chest level. Count to 10 or take 3 to 5 deep breaths.
Come out of the pose and repeat it on the other side. You'll
feel fabulous. Don't get confused with left and right as you
do the pose on the other side.

warrior III

This pose stretches the spine and strengthens the leg muscles, feet and toes.

Do this pose when you're feeling unclear or indecisive and it'll help you balance your choices.

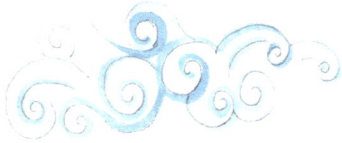

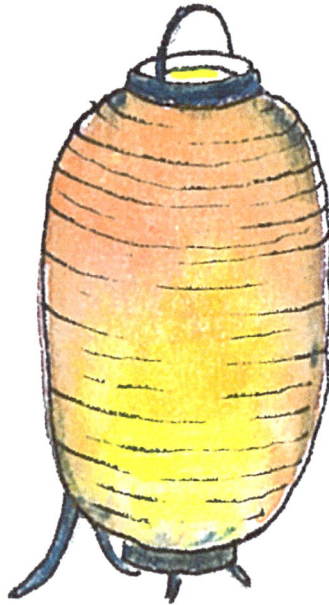

ZEN POINT

Sometimes it feels like you're all on your own when you believe in something others cannot imagine. Don't be afraid of that feeling, and keep your dreams alive.

MINDFUL FACT

Do balancing poses with your eyes open.

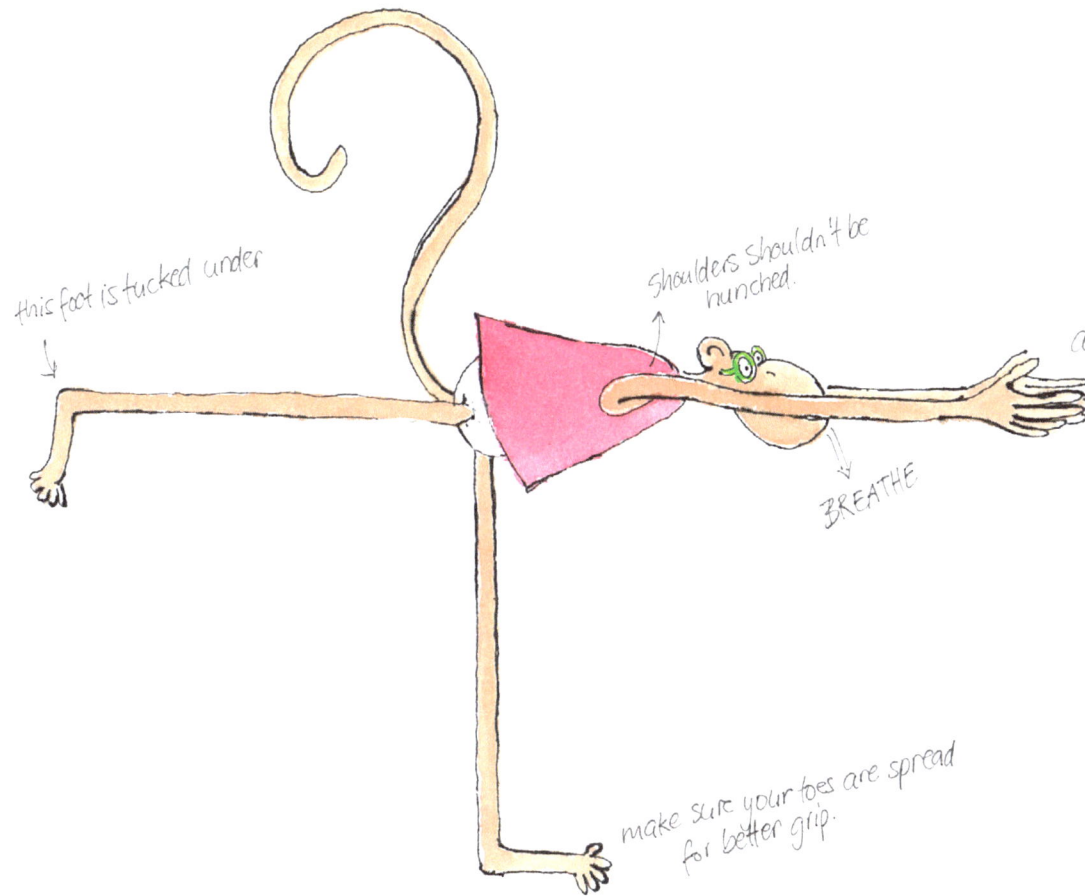

this foot is tucked under

Shoulders shouldn't be hunched.

arms parallel palms facing each other.

BREATHE

make sure your toes are spread for better grip.

1

2

Start from standing mountain pose and plant the standing leg firmly on the floor. Bring your arms up as if you're going to do upward facing salute but don't overreach. Now tilt forward from the hips without bending your spine. It doesn't matter how low you can bend as long as there is a straight line from the tips of your fingers back to your heel.

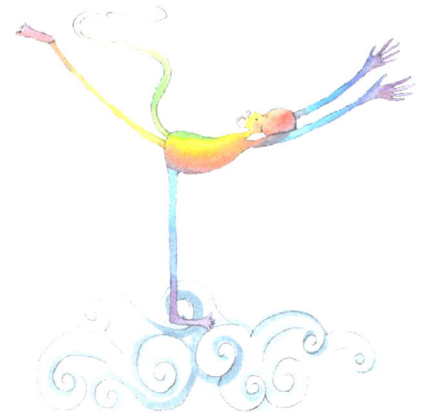

Hold the pose and breathe. Maybe you can stretch your leg even higher. Try! Stretch your chest and reach up. This is quite a challenge. "Wahoo! This is like flying." Gently come out of the pose and try the other leg. Remember, drop the monkey mind and concentrate on balance.

crescent moon pose

This pose makes you strong and balanced. It opens the heart and it will bring creativity to the right side of the brain and let the tired, logical left side, often strained with cold facts, rest.

This is one of Aristotle's favourite poses.

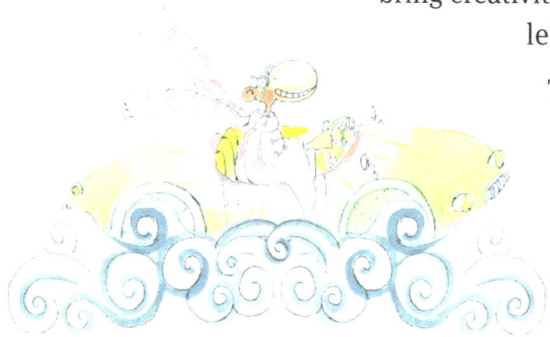

Perhaps not every lunatic is mad. Maybe he's just ticking in time with the moon cycle. We all go a bit loony sometimes, especially around full-moon time.

Reminder: genius is akin to madness.

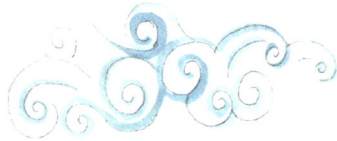

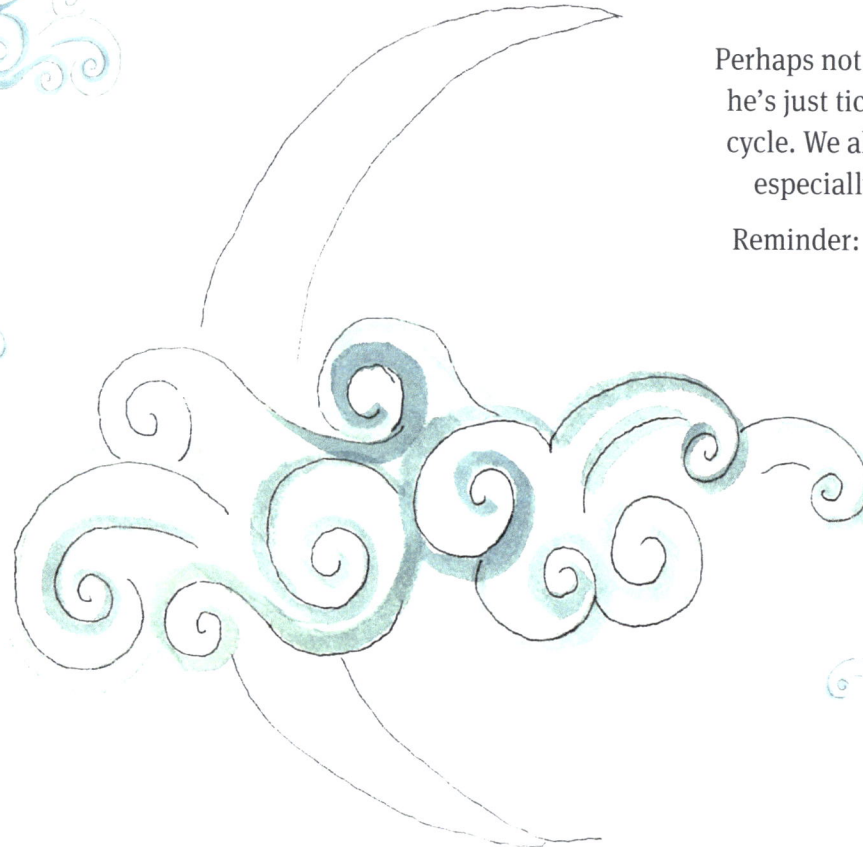

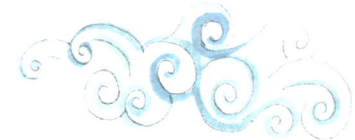

The moon shines even if its face is covered by clouds. Try to imagine you're like the moon even if it feels like the clouds are taking over.

1

breathe

tilt at the hips into warrior III

plant your standing leg firmly into the ground

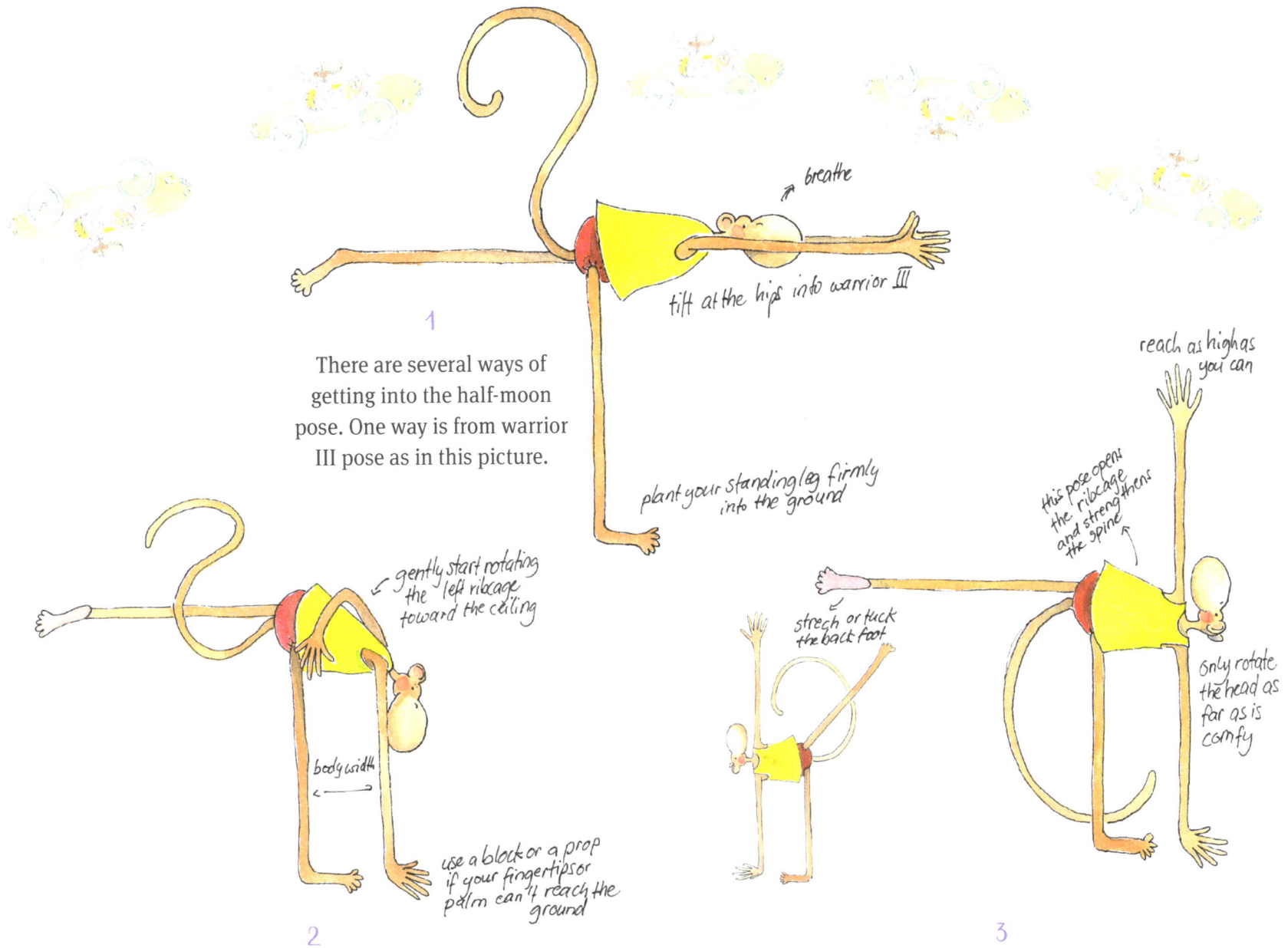

There are several ways of getting into the half-moon pose. One way is from warrior III pose as in this picture.

2

gently start rotating the left ribcage toward the ceiling

body width

use a block or a prop if your fingertips or palm can't reach the ground

Now place the right hand in front of the right foot at body-width distance. Rest the left arm on the left hip. Breathe! Now rotate your hips and heart to the left side.

3

reach as high as you can

this pose opens the ribcage and strengthens the spine

stretch or tuck the back foot

only rotate the head as far as is comfy

Lift your left arm up toward the ceiling and look at your thumb. If you lose your balance, try again, and again, and again . . . stay in the moment. Don't judge yourself if your balance isn't quite there yet. Count to 10 or take 5 even breaths. Smile! Do the other side now.

tree pose

Tones the muscles in the legs and brings balance to the mind and spirit. Caution point—the bending leg foot should not rest on the knee joint, as this causes unnecessary pressure on the joint.

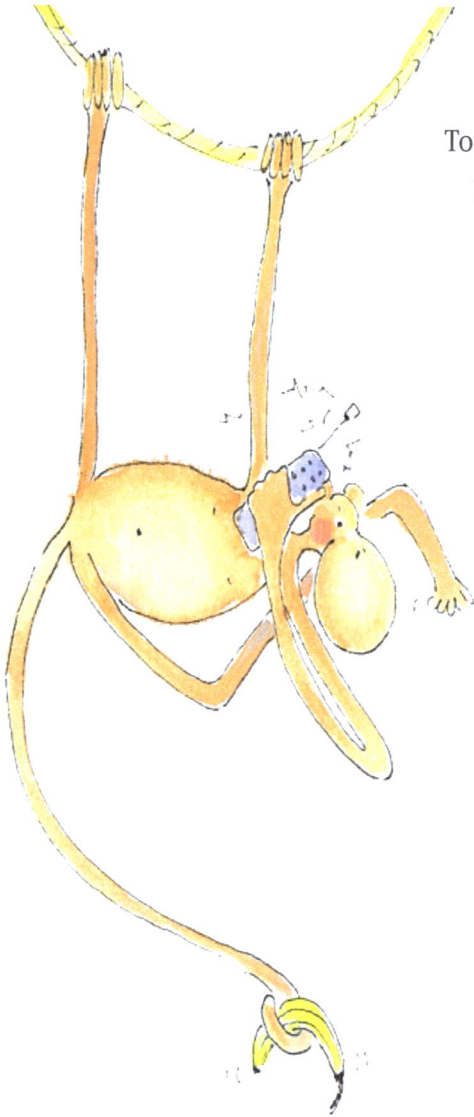

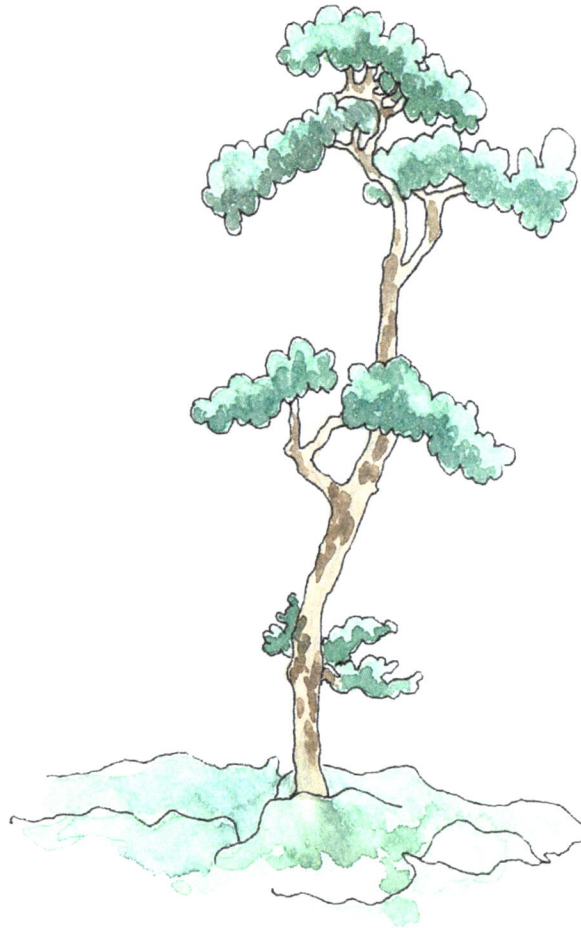

ZEN POINT

THE WORLD IS LIKE A MIRROR, YOU SEE? SMILE AND YOUR FRIENDS SMILE BACK.

- JAPANESE PROVERB

Yoga is like a tree with 8 main branches.
Postures are the third branch of the 8-branched yoga tree.
Keep a pure mind and heart and all else will follow.

This pose is so much fun
concentrate and breathe

remember to
do the pose on both sides

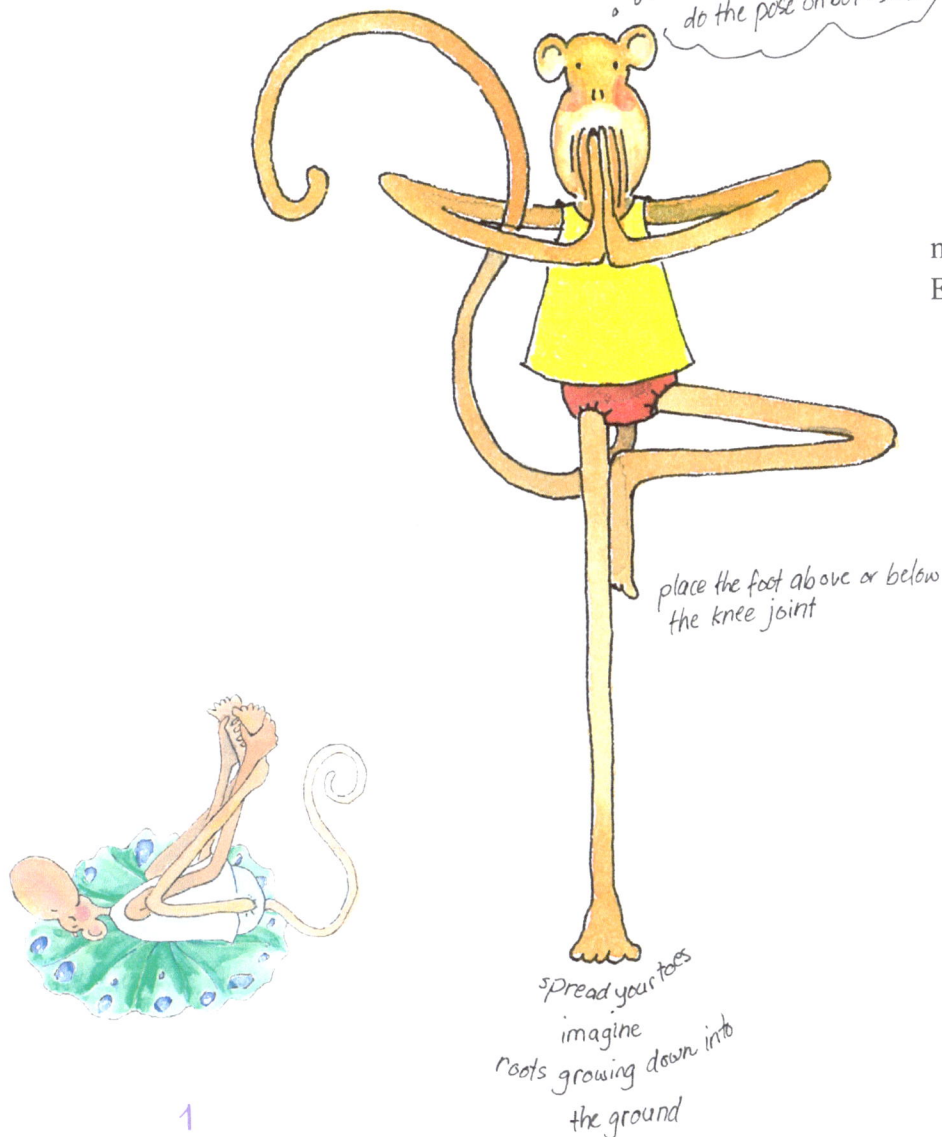

MINDFUL FACT

Exercise brings circulation to the whole body:
the feet, the bones, the muscles, the skin, the
nails and hair, the heart and lungs and the brain.
Exercise helps concentration and understanding.
This will help you with your homework.

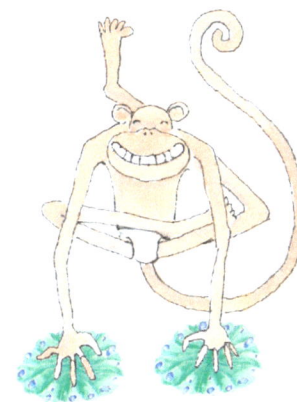

place the foot above or below
the knee joint

spread your toes
imagine
roots growing down into
the ground

1

2

First make sure your feet are firmly planted on the mat. Choose
a leg to stand on and then grab your other leg at the ankle and
press the foot into the inner thigh of the opposite standing leg.

Bring your hands to your heart. "Namaste." Count to 10 or take 5
deep breaths (Aristotle likes to stay in this pose for a good minute),
focus and balance. Now repeat the pose on the other standing leg.

head-to-knee pose

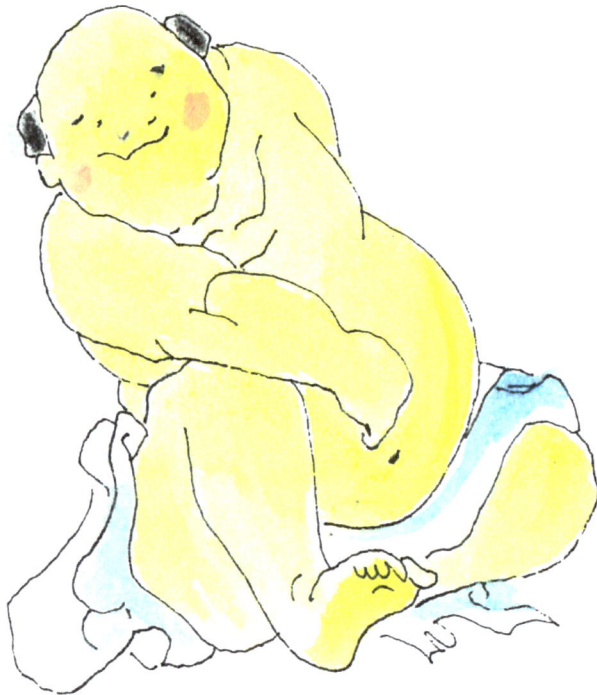

BAND AID/LIVE AID/LIVE 8

In 1985—Building on the momentum of Band Aid, dual Live Aid concerts were held in London and Philadelphia on 13 July. Over a billion and a half people worldwide watched the 16-hour event on television, in which over 60 of the biggest stars in rock music performed, and over £100 million was raised for African famine relief. Musical and political history was made.

In 2005—Bob Geldof organised the Live 8 concerts for third world debt relief:

"THIS IS NOT LIVE AID 2. THESE CONCERTS ARE THE STARTING POINT FOR THE LONG WALK TO JUSTICE, THE ONE WAY WE CAN ALL MAKE OUR VOICES HEARD IN UNISON."

- BOB GELDOF

How about raising money through a worldwide yoga event to help save our environment?

David Williams, the famous Ashtanga yoga teacher, tells us to make yoga a 50-year goal. There is no rush, keep trying a little bit every day.

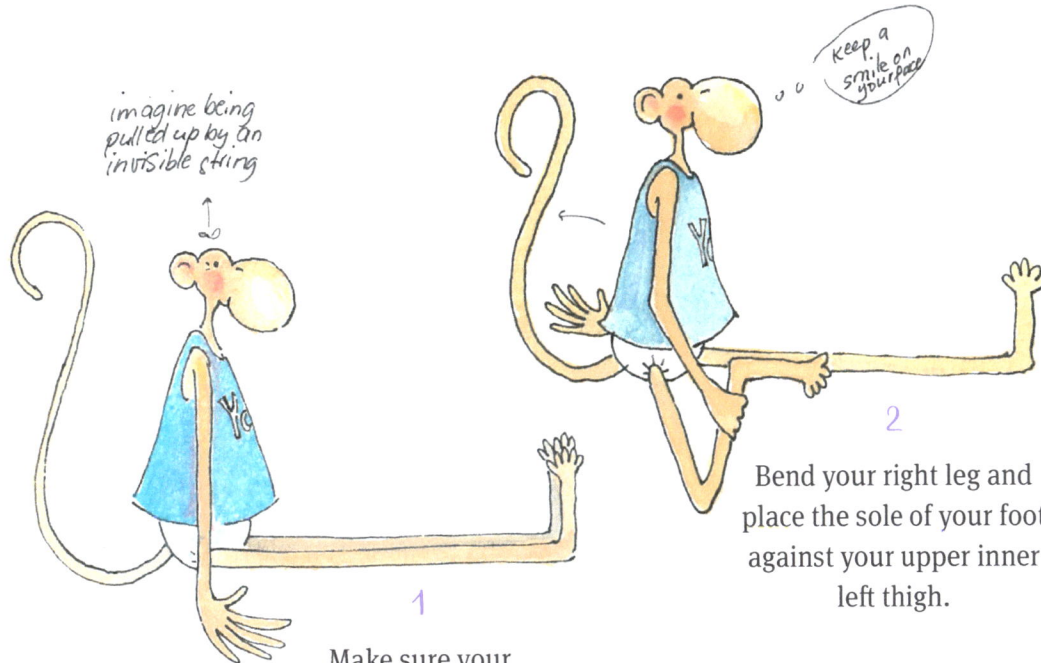

imagine being pulled up by an invisible string

Keep a smile on your face

the turtle, not the rabbit wins the race

if you cannot reach the foot grab the ankle

1
Make sure your bottom is firmly planted on the mat.

2
Bend your right leg and place the sole of your foot against your upper inner left thigh.

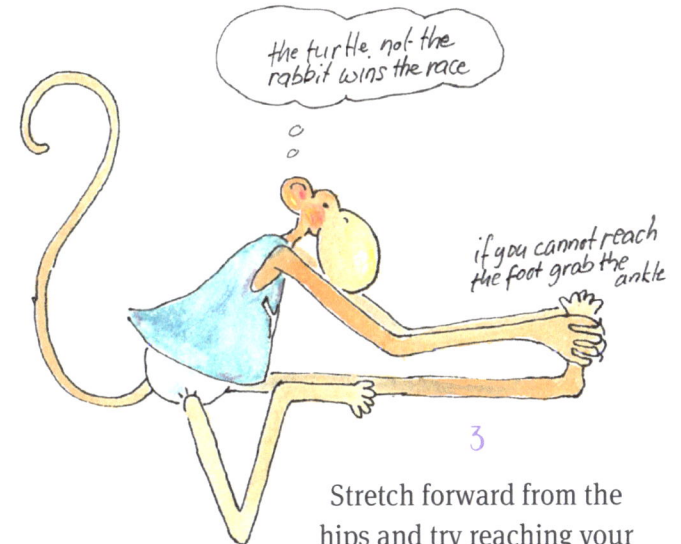

3
Stretch forward from the hips and try reaching your ankle or toes. Breathe.

Oh, this side is a bit more difficult...

repeat steps 1 to 4 3 times

count to 10 ... and feel the gentle pull at the back of your knee

This pose is good for your organs. According to Geeta Iyengar's instructions, in case of persistent low fever, this pose should be performed on each side for 5 minutes.

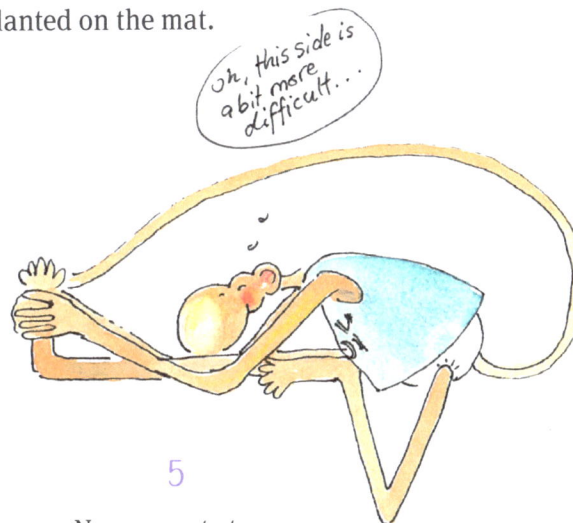

5
Now repeat steps 1 to 4 bending the opposite leg.

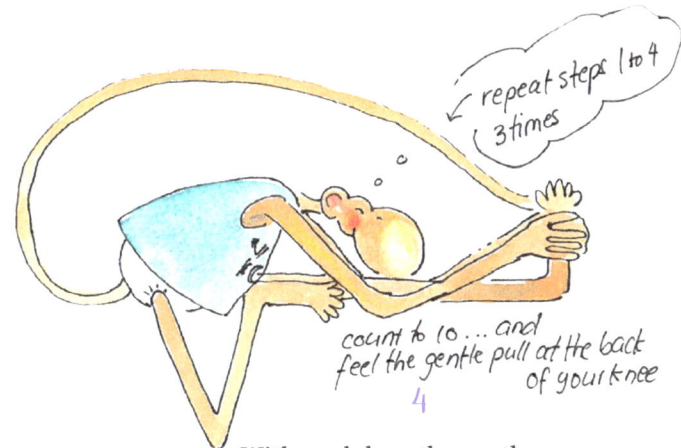

4
With each breath, gently come lower toward your leg. Take long slow breaths.

boat pose

This pose brings relief and vigour to the back
and strengthens the belly.

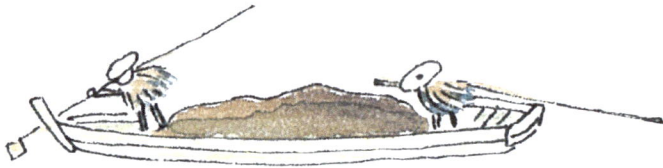

Play a game of yoga tag with your
friends. The person being tagged has
to stand in triangle, warrior I or II
pose, or downward-facing dog until
someone slides through and
underneath the pose and you're freed.
This is fun and gets you breathing.

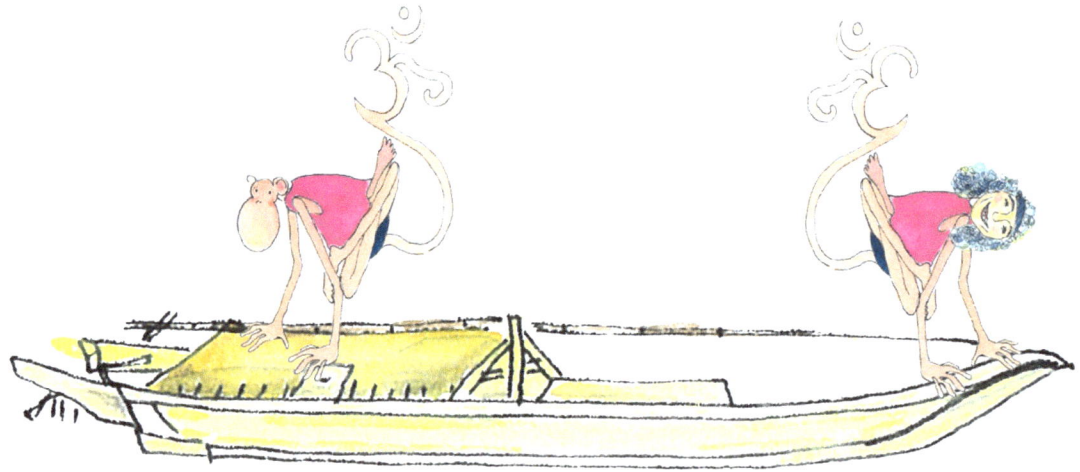

ZEN POINT

If you don't really need something,
simply say, "I have enough, thank
you." That way we won't waste so
many of our natural resources.

♡ 50 ♡

This pose can get a bit wiggly

Oops! I can hardly breathe from concentrating

2

Keep your back straight. Start lifting your legs. Breath gently.

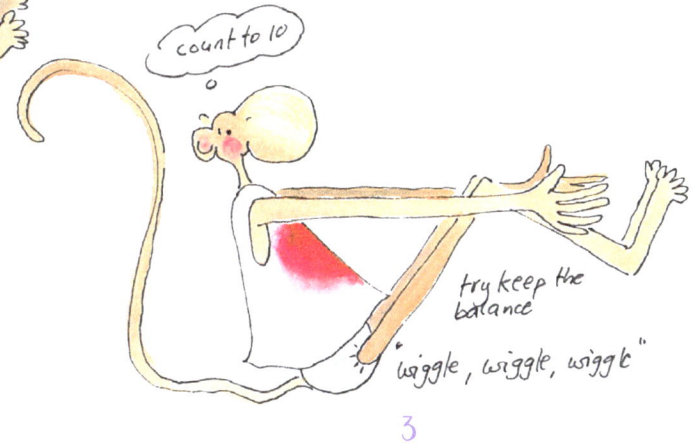

count to 10

try keep the balance

"wiggle, wiggle, wiggle"

3

Now, stretch your arms out parallel to the floor, arms facing each other. Stay in this pose for 3 to 5 long in and out breaths.

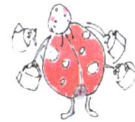

Well done everyone!

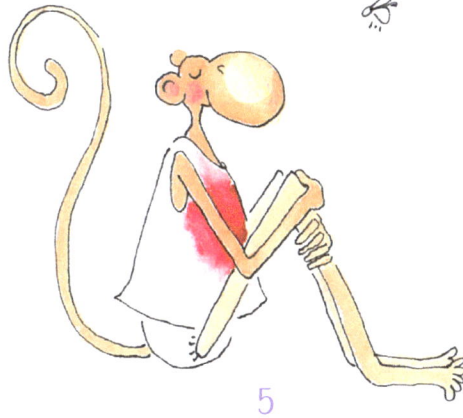

1

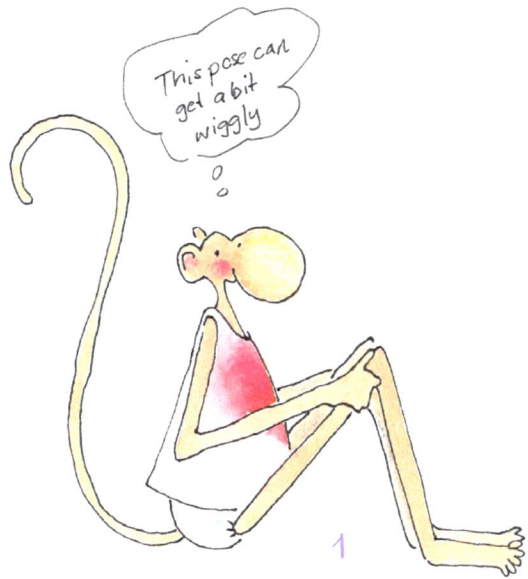

Sit on the floor with your bottom firmly in place and your knees tucked in.

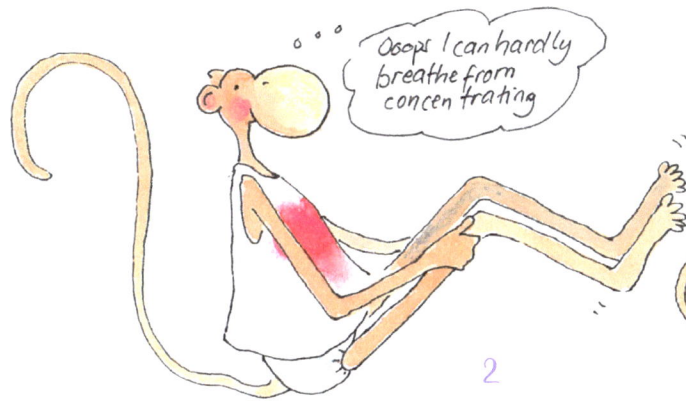

focus on your toes

your tummy muscles will get stronger

5

Finally come back out of the pose. Close your eyes and give your knees a hug. Repeat steps 1 to 5 three times.

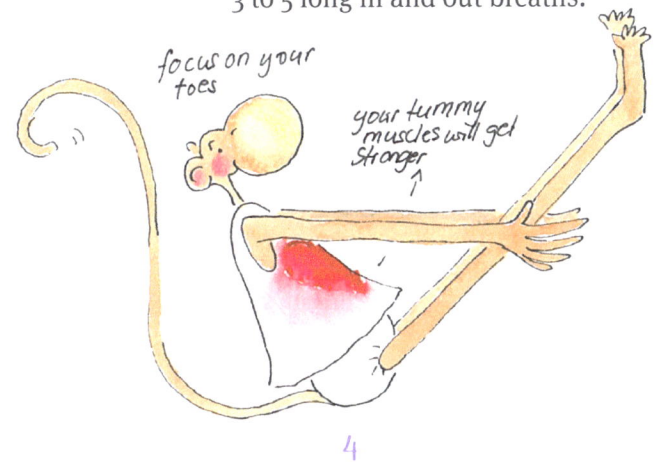

4

Once your strength is built in your belly, see if you can straighten the legs. Wow!

lotus pose

Populations of many species, from fish to mammals, have dropped because of human threats such as pollution, clearing of forests and overfishing.

Everything is connected. We depend on nature.

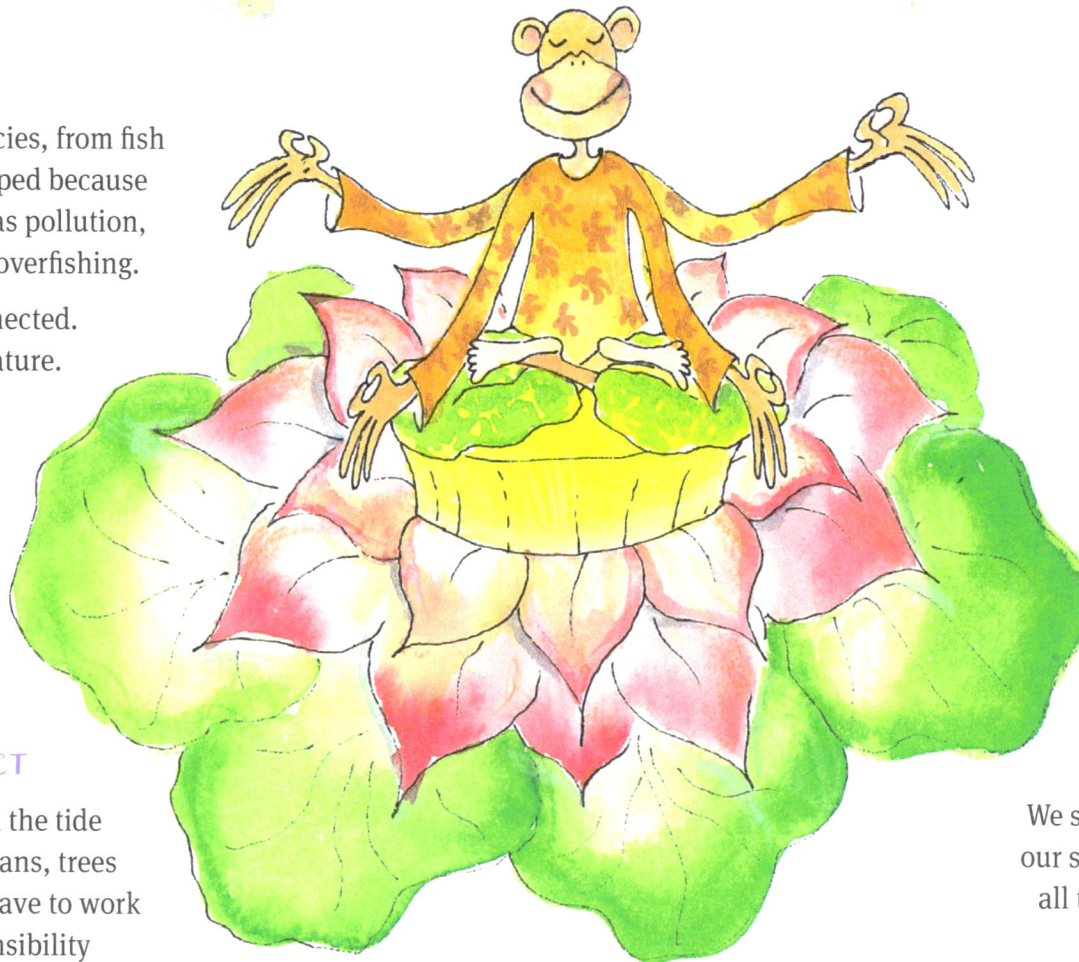

MINDFUL FACT

It's not too late to turn the tide around, to save our oceans, trees and animals, but we all have to work it out and take responsibility together now, today.

ZEN POINT

We sit on nature, nature is our supportive seat. We are all the custodians of our earth.

1

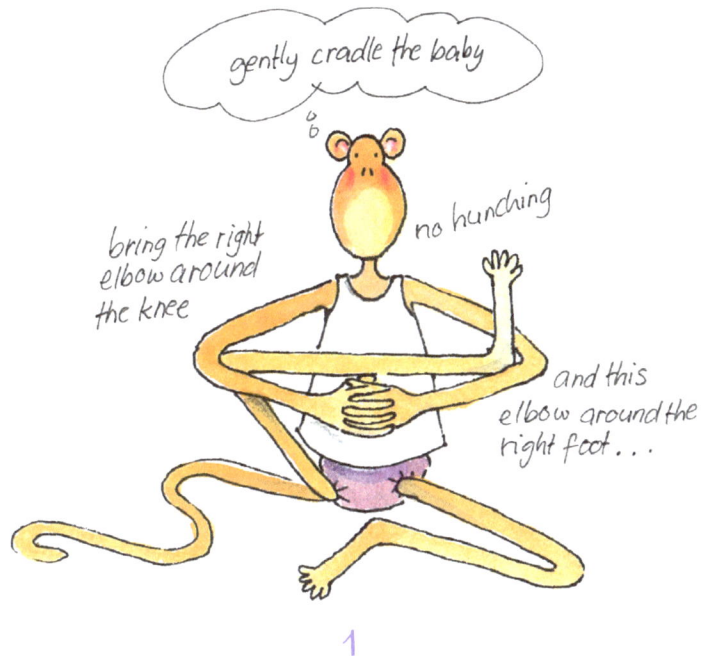

First, sit in a simple cross-legged pose. Then, take one leg and cradle it like a baby.

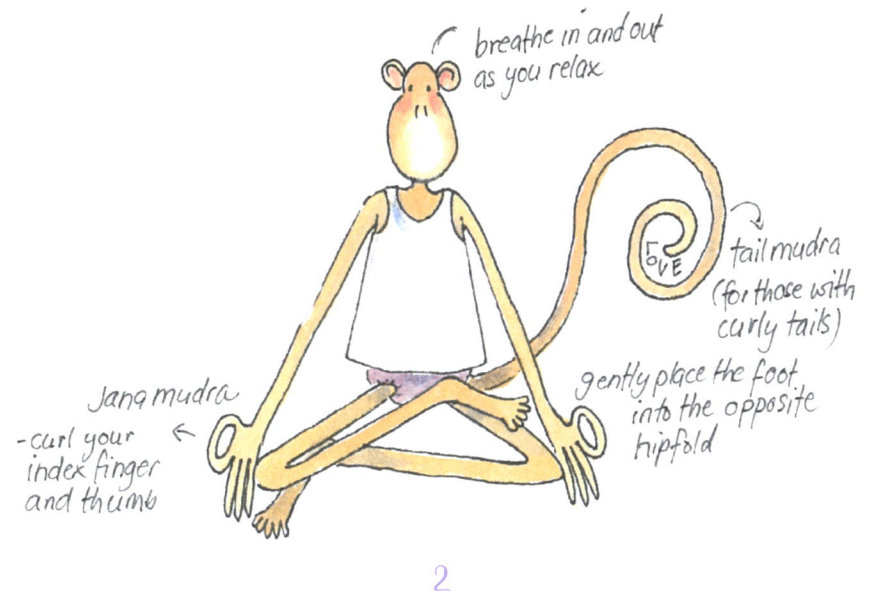

2

See if you can rest that foot on your opposite thigh. This is half-lotus pose.

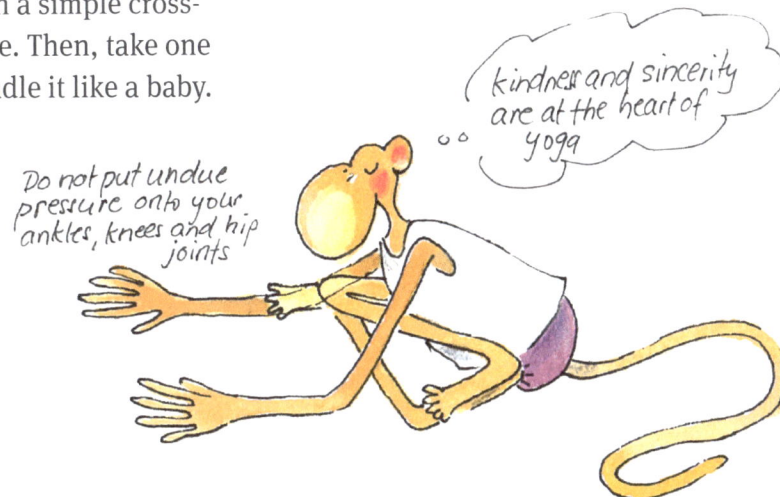

3

Now, if this feels comfortable, gently bend forward and breathe.

Now repeat the above steps with the other leg.

grasshopper pose followed by bow pose

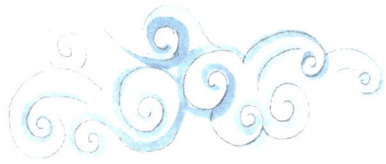

This pose really strengthens your back, bottom and legs. It opens the chest and also helps massage the inside of your belly.

Remember don't do yoga after eating a big meal.

ZEN POINT

YOU ARE THE BOW, YOUR CHILDREN THE ARROW. A GOOD PARENT IS IN TUNE WITH THE WAY THE ARROW IS POSITIONED SO IT CAN SOAR . . .

– KATRINA KENISON, ROLF GATES, MEDITATION FROM THE MAT

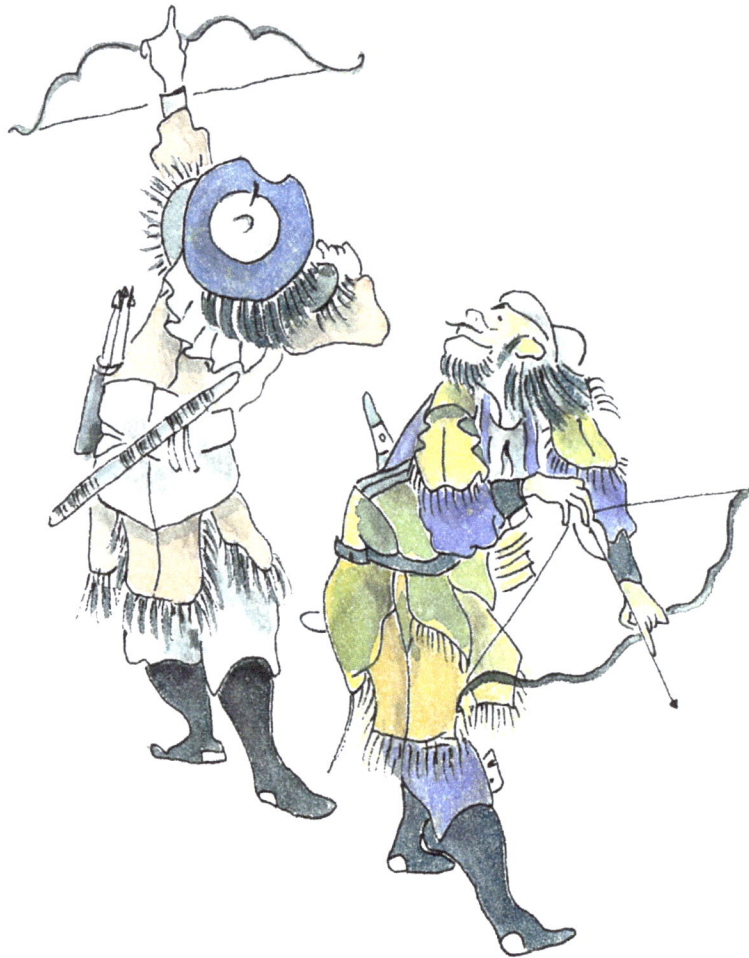

MINDFUL FACT

Your body is the bow and your arms are the string, your heart is the arrow.

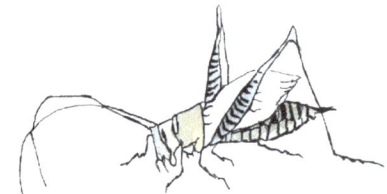

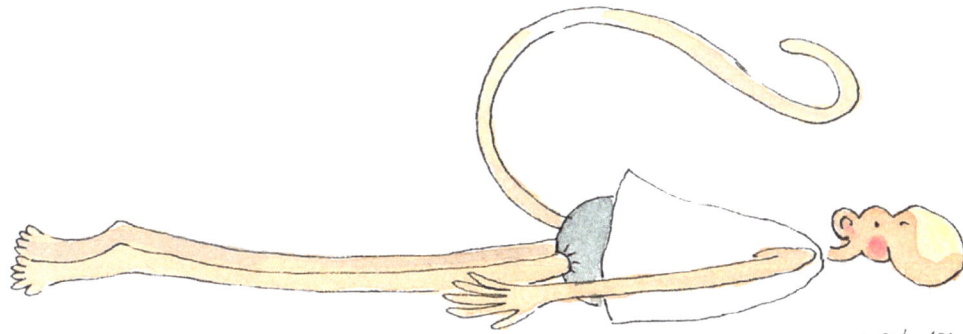

palms face down

rest your chin or
forehead on the mat

1

Lie on your belly with your arms
next to your body.

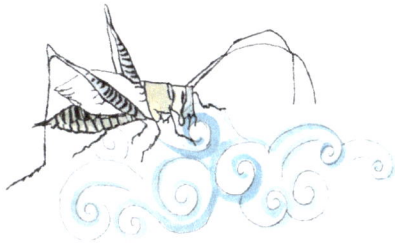

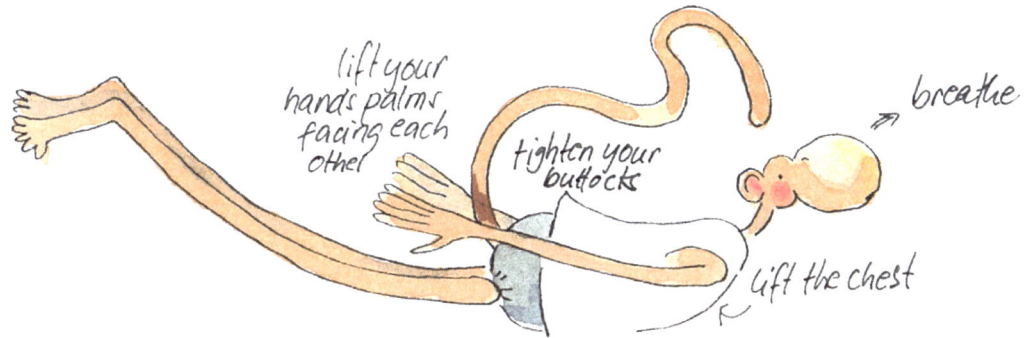

lift your
hand's palms
facing each
other

tighten your
buttocks

breathe

lift the chest

2

Now tighten your buttocks and thigh muscles and
slowly lift your upper body, legs and arms off the
floor into grasshopper pose. Take 5 deep breaths.
Rest in position 3.

3

Haaa "rest between the pose

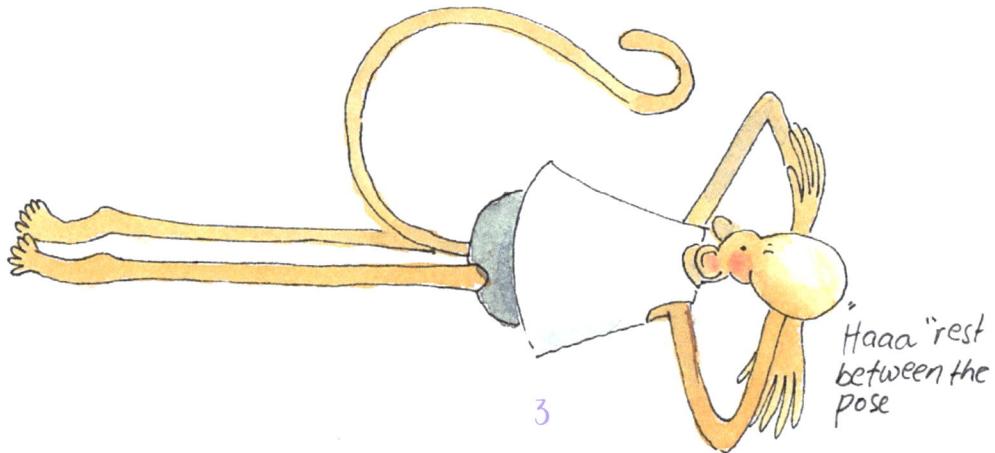

Let the creative energy
fill your body.

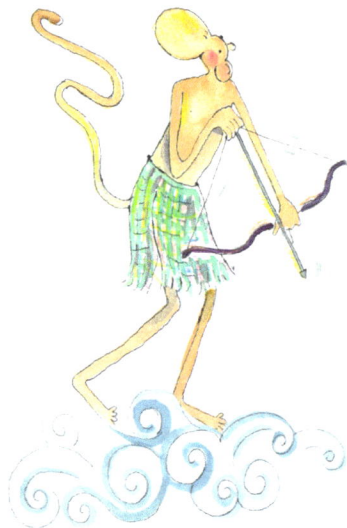

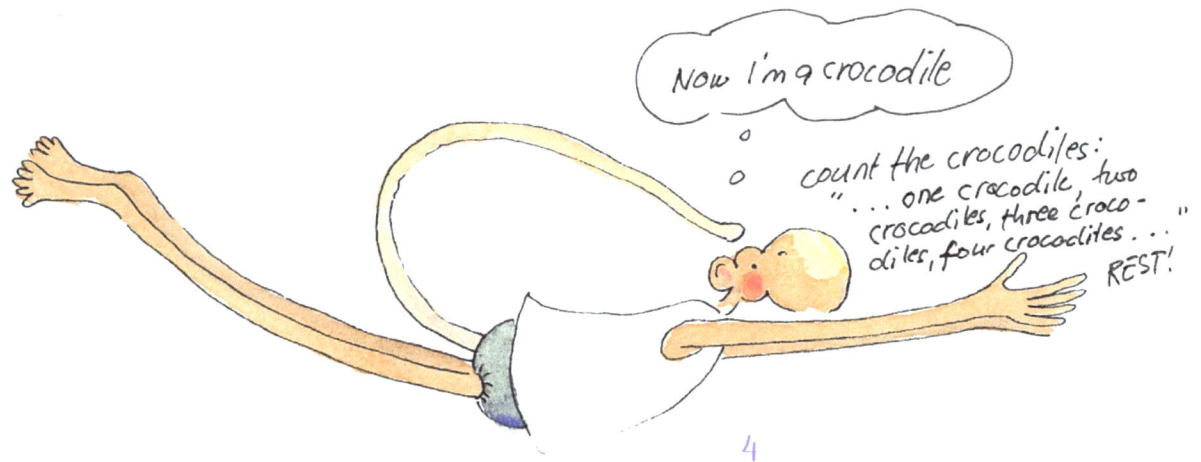

Now I'm a crocodile

count the crocodiles:
"... one crocodile, two
crocodiles, three croco-
diles, four crocodiles ..."
REST!

4

After your break, instead of stretching the arms
behind you as in grasshopper pose, lift and extend
them forward in front of you in crocodile pose. Take 5
breaths and rest in position 3 before trying position 5.

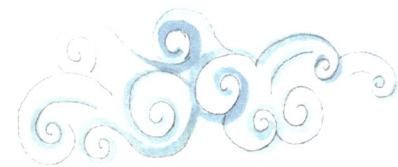

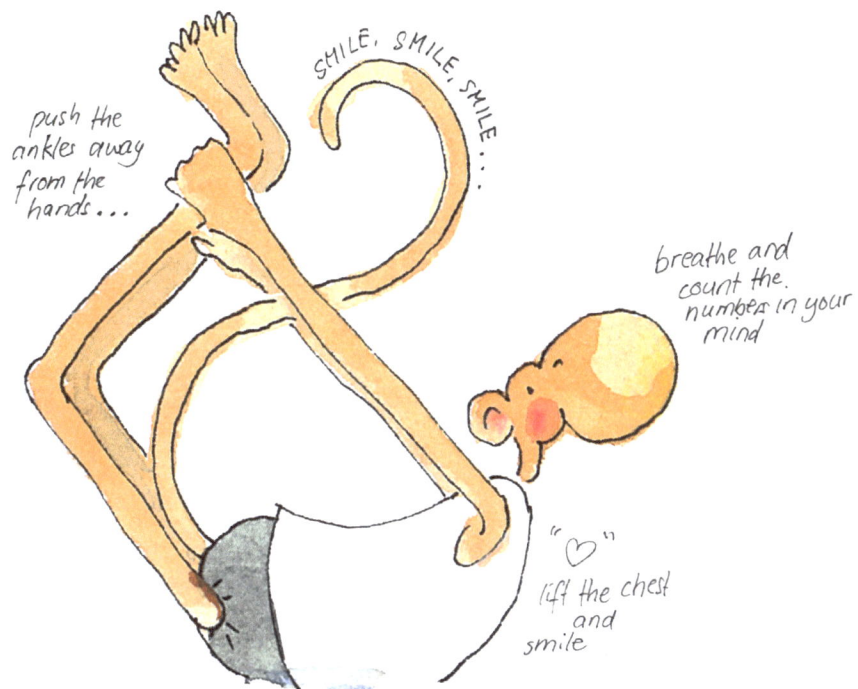

push the
ankles away
from the
hands...

SMILE, SMILE, SMILE...

breathe and
count the
numbers in your
mind

"♡"
lift the chest
and
smile

5

Now try bow pose. Push those heels away into your
hands and count to 10. Don't forget to breathe.

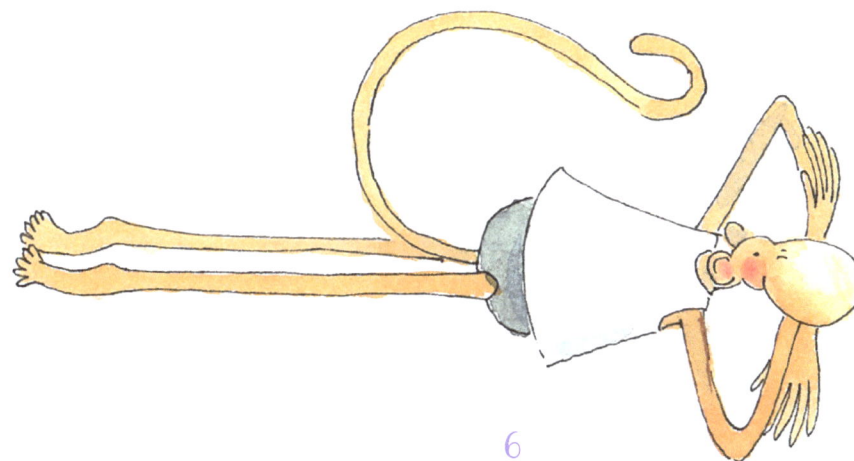

6

Let the creative energy fill your body
and repeat bow pose 2 more times.

turtle pose

This pose calms your nerves and brings balance to your emotions.
Start off gently.

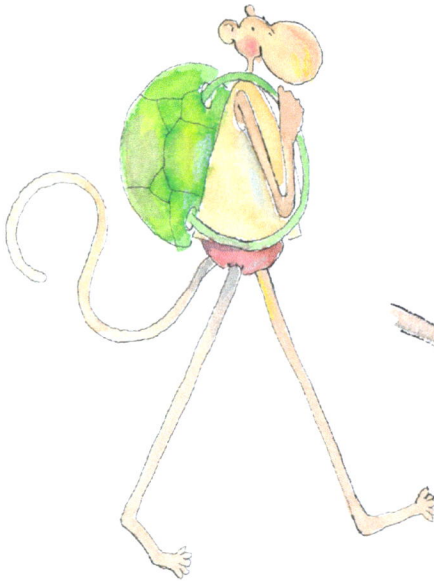

MINDFUL FACT

OBESITY IS THE WORLD'S FASTEST
GROWING HEALTH PROBLEM.

ZEN POINT

The tortoise not the hare wins the race. Do a
little bit of yoga every day. Start with sitting
quietly, then breathe and stretch in cat pose
and downward-facing dog pose. Now repeat 5
sun salutations, sit for twenty-five breaths in
half lotus on both sides . . . then jump under
a blanket and rest for 10 minutes. Yummy.

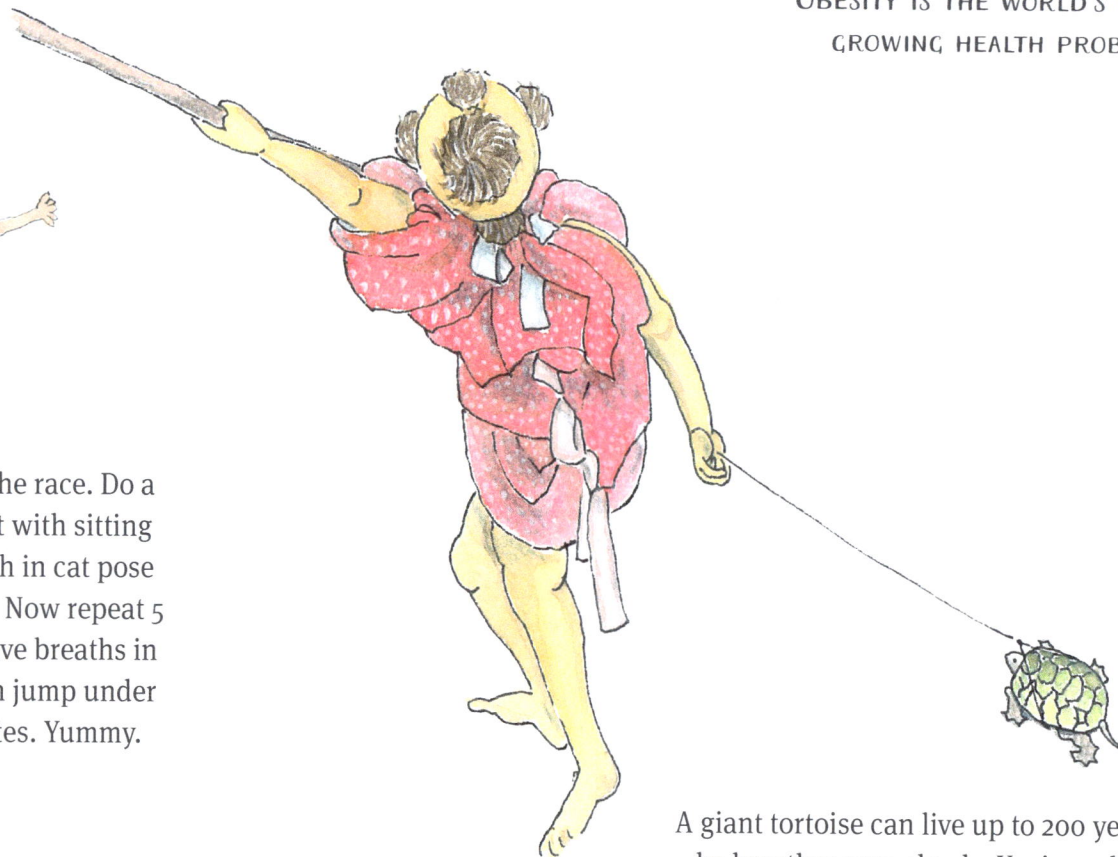

A giant tortoise can live up to 200 years because she/
he breathes very slowly. Yogis understood that by
consciously pacing the breath one can live longer.
Don't waste your breath unnecessarily.

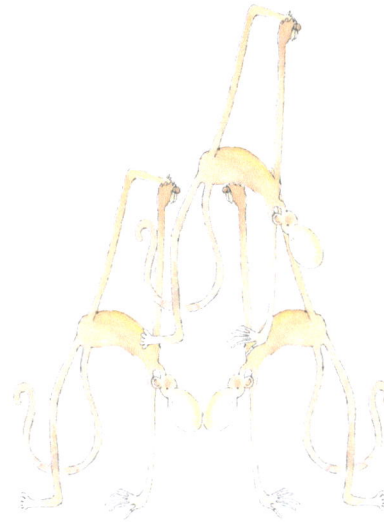

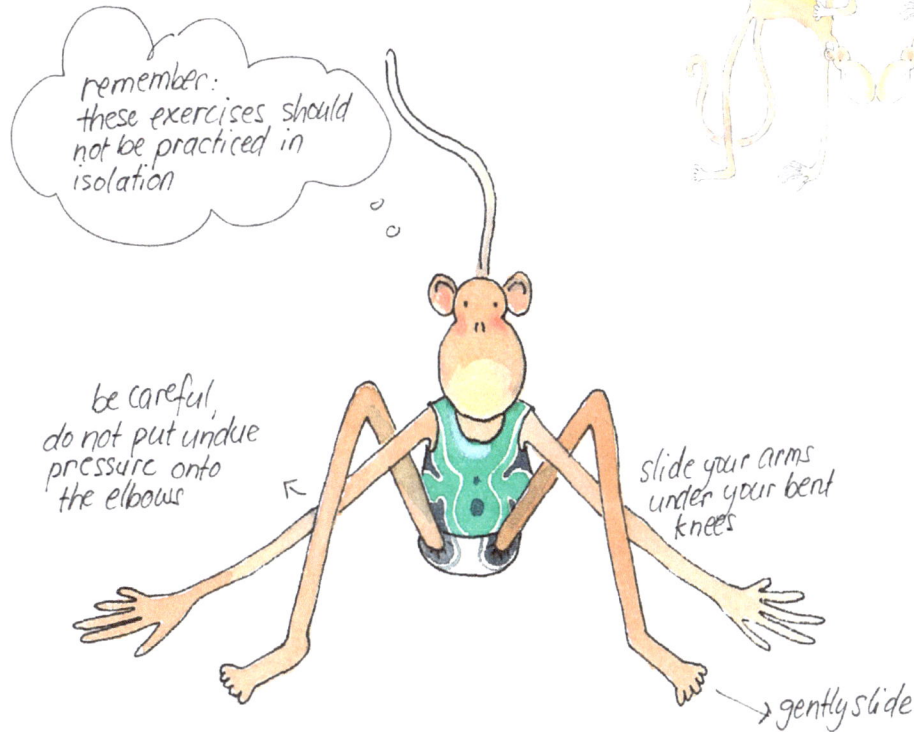

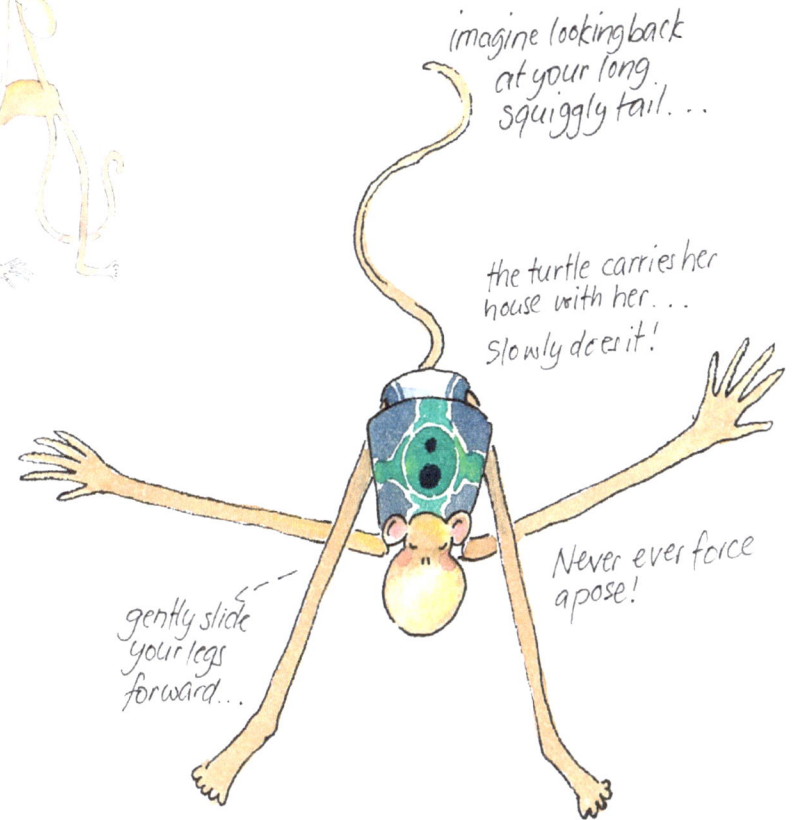

1

Sit on the floor with your legs spread and your knees bent as in the picture. Slip your arms under the knees and take a deep breath.

2

Slowly start sliding your legs forward as far as is comfortably possible for you. It takes time until you are able to get the shoulders to rest on the floor, so don't push it. Breathe deeply and evenly. Never force a pose.

wheel pose

Keeps the body supple and alert and makes you feel energetic,
light and alive. It also reduces the fat around the waist.

ZEN POINT

Eat more vegetables, rice and beans
and less sweet and salty snacks. Have
porridge with fruit for breakfast and try
not to eat after 8 o'clock in the evening.

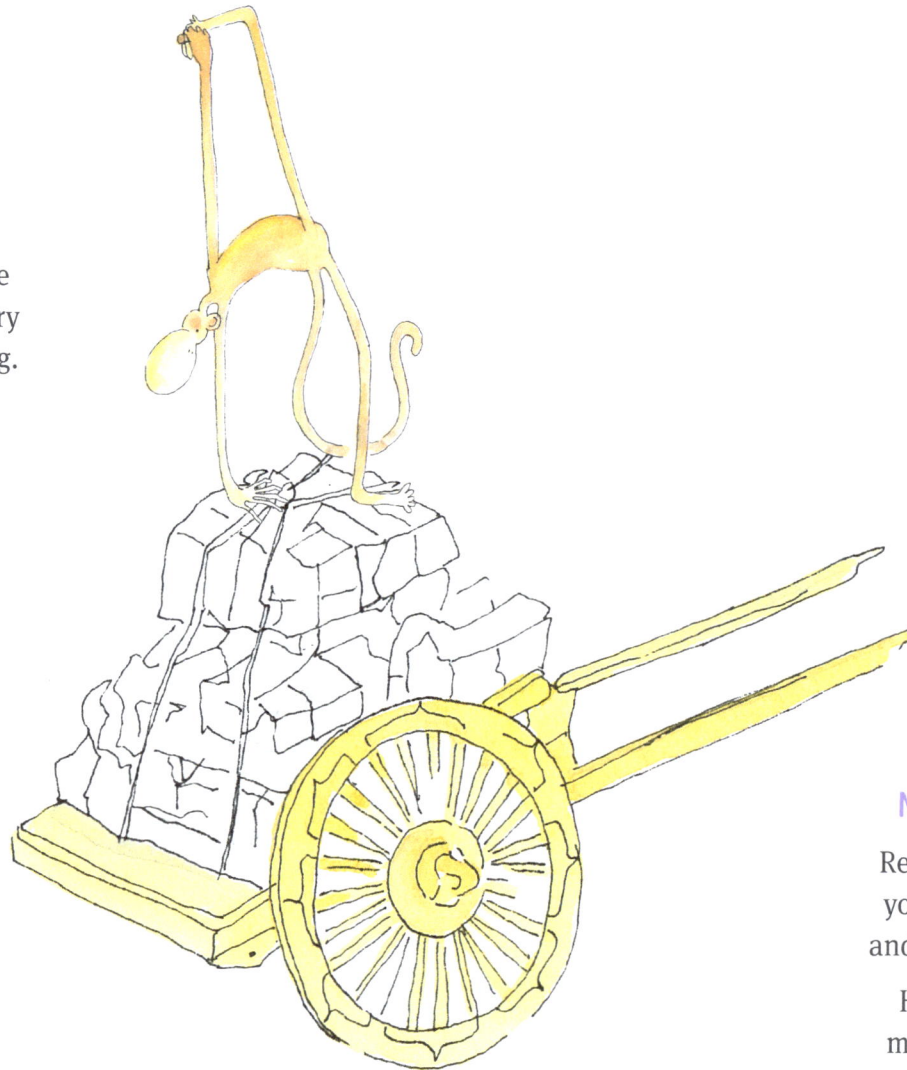

MINDFUL FACT

Regular exercise puts
you in a better mood
and keeps you healthy.

Healthy heart and
mind, healthy body.

knees are parallel

elbows are shoulder-width apart

1

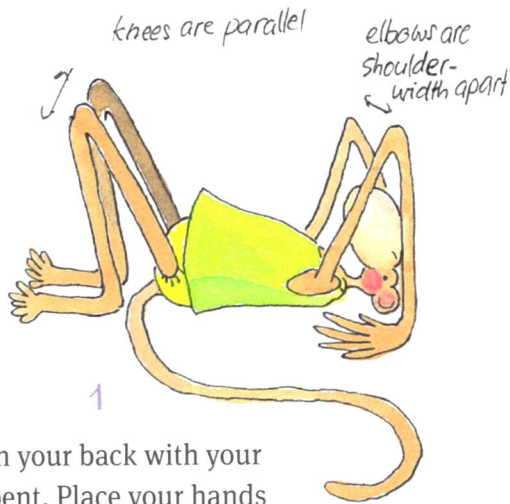

Lie on your back with your legs bent. Place your hands behind your shoulders.

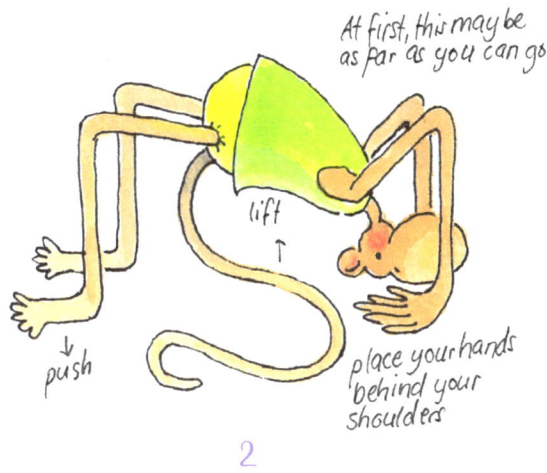

At first, this may be as far as you can go

lift

push

place your hands behind your shoulders

2

Breathe in and if you can't come into position 3, try to come onto the crown of your head without putting too much pressure on your neck.

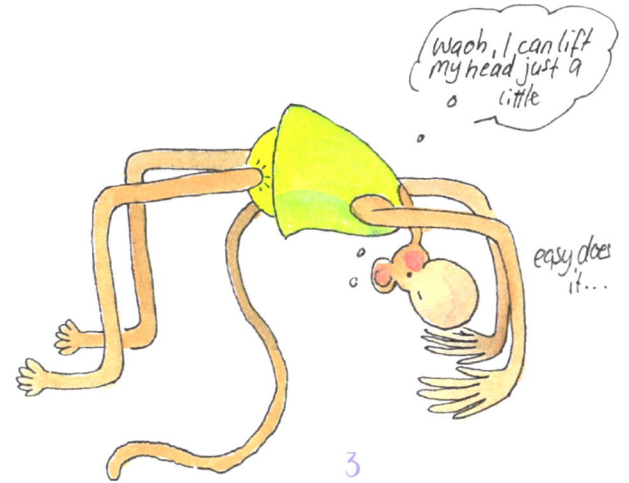

Waoh, I can lift my head just a little

easy does it...

3

As you get stronger you'll be able to lift the head off the mat.

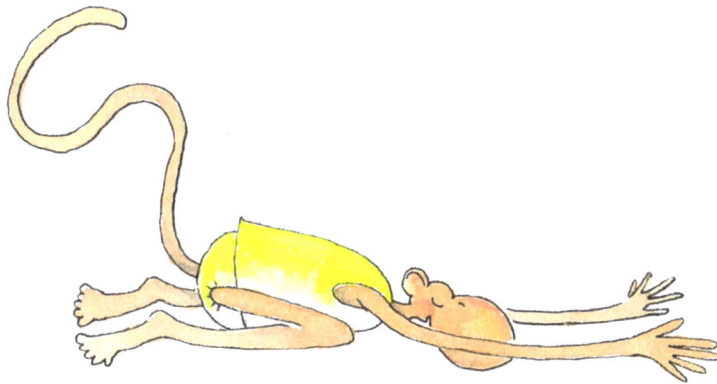

open your upper back

breathe 3 to 6 in and out breaths

4

Now stretch your arms and start lifting your head off the mat. Take 5 breaths. Carefully come down and give your knees a cuddle. You can try the same pose 2 more times.

5

Then rest in child's pose. You deserve it!

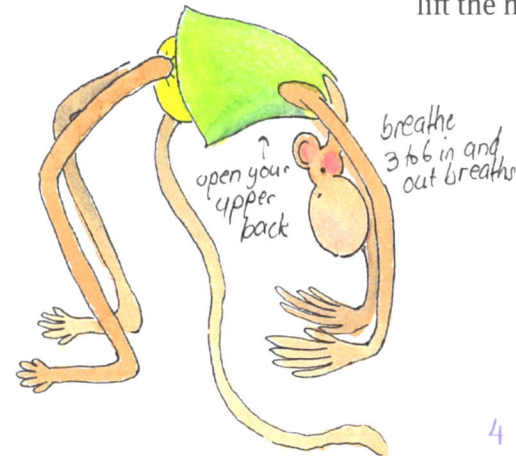

seated forward bend

Bends are soothing, calming and lengthen the entire back side of your body. They improve circulation, and nourish and heal your frayed nerves.

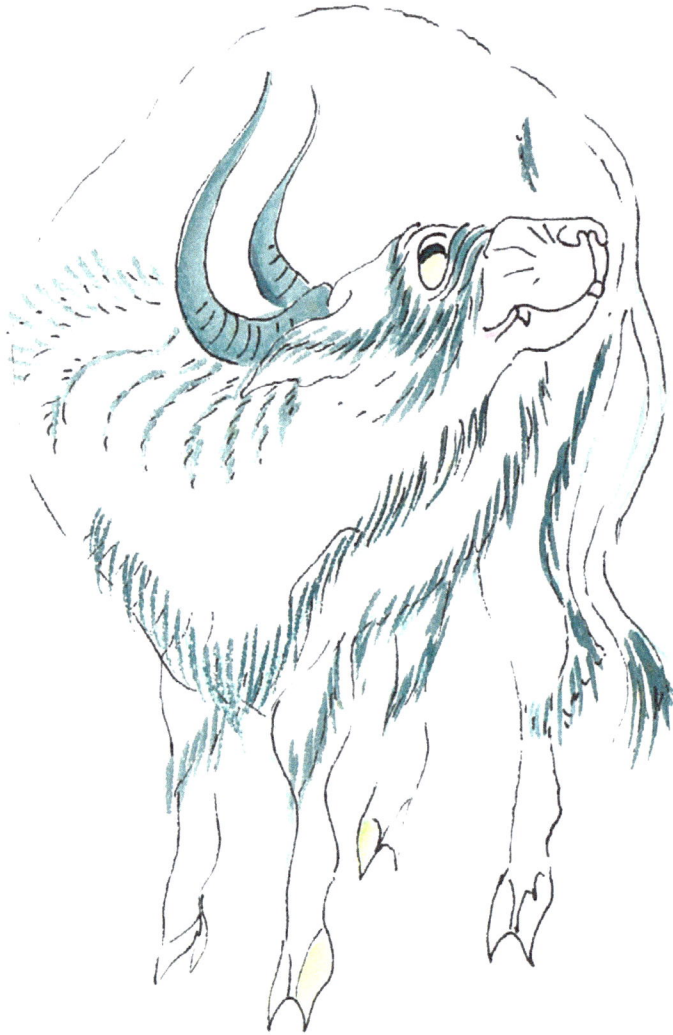

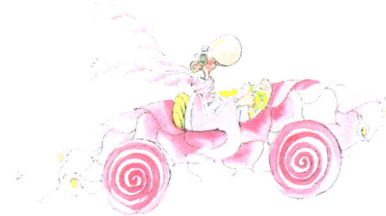

MINDFUL FACT

TV, CDs, DVDs AND COMPUTER GAMES ARE FUN FOR MOST CHILDREN. THERE IS NO REASON WHY THEY SHOULDN'T BE ENTERTAINED IN THIS WAY SOME OF THE TIME. TOO MUCH TIME IN FRONT OF A SCREEN, HOWEVER, CAN CREATE A PASSIVE, INACTIVE CHILD. THE ISSUE BECOMES ONE OF BALANCE.

- ANDY GRIFFITHS, JIM THOMSON, SOPHIE BLACKMORE, "FAST FOOD AND NO PLAY MAKE JACK A FAT BOY" (2005)

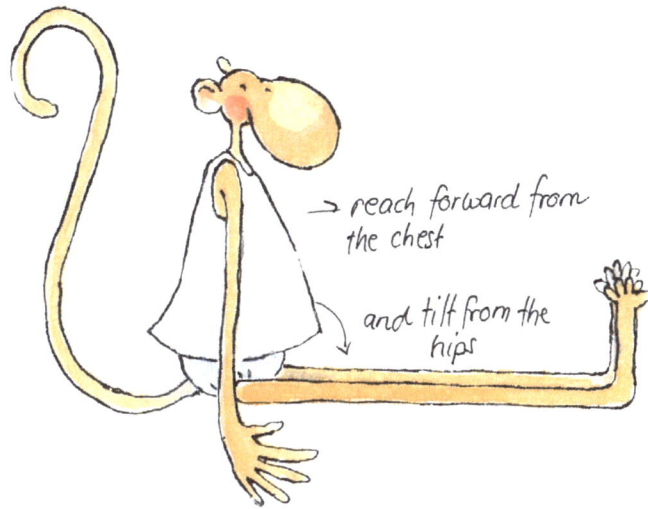

reach forward from the chest

and tilt from the hips

1

Sit on your bottom, with legs in front of you.

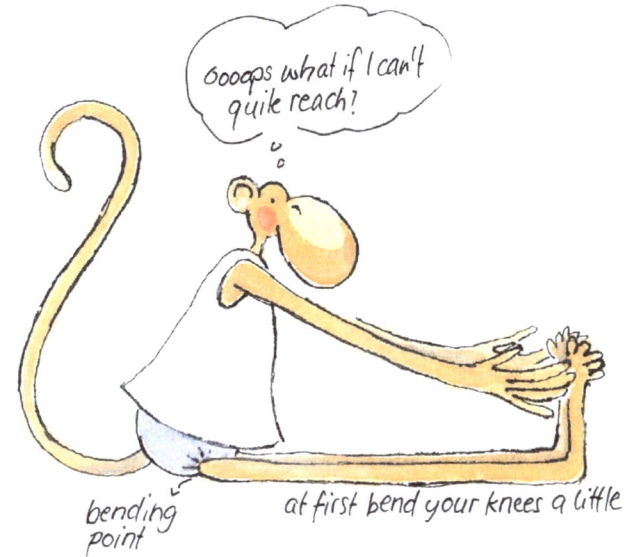

oooops what if I can't quite reach!

bending point

at first bend your knees a little

2

Gently bend forward and try not to hunch your shoulders.

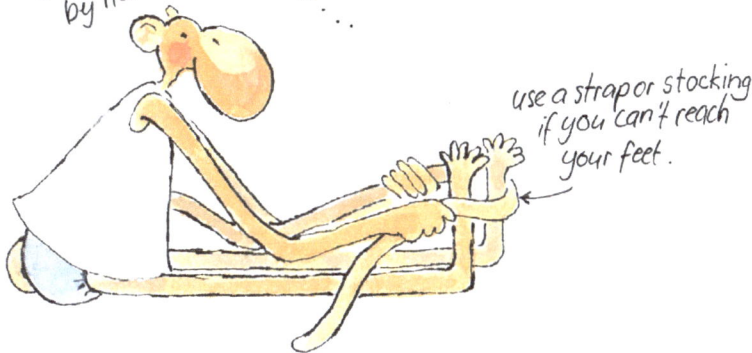

don't compromise the stretch by hunching shoulders...

use a strap or stocking if you can't reach your feet.

3

Use a long sock, or stocking like Pippi Longstocking, or strap to help reach if your arms feel too short. Breathe deeply and with each outbreath relax more into the pose.

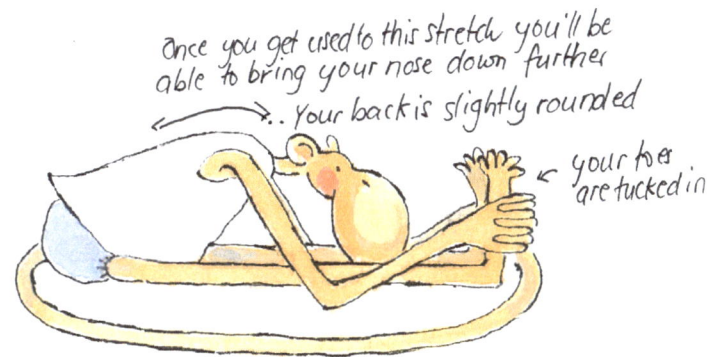

once you get used to this stretch you'll be able to bring your nose down further

..Your back is slightly rounded

your toes are tucked in

4

With practice, everything will start to fall into the right place. Keep going and surprise yourself. It's important to stay joyful. Count to 10 and rest before trying 2 more times.

rabbit pose

To avoid injury whilst shifting weight onto the head, you can keep your hands on the floor next to your shoulders until you feel safe.

This is a great pose. It opens and strengthens the chest and helps you find inner balance when turning upside down.

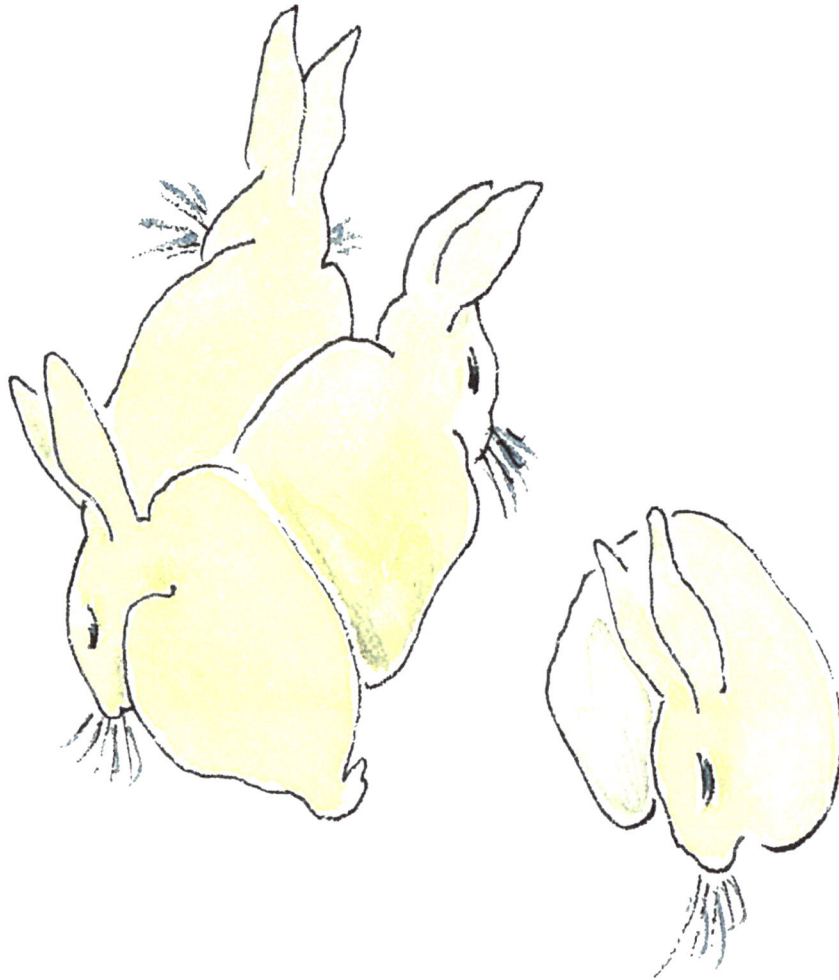

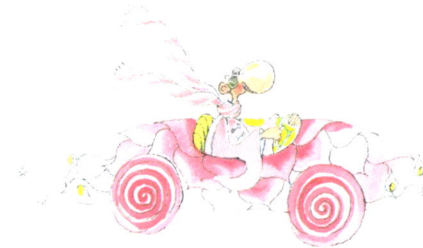

this pose is like child's pose ... then you activate your arms...

interlock your fingers and stretch your arms high

1

Come forward and down into child's pose as in the picture, interlock your hands behind your back and lift them up as high as possible. Breathe. This is a biiiiiiig stretch!

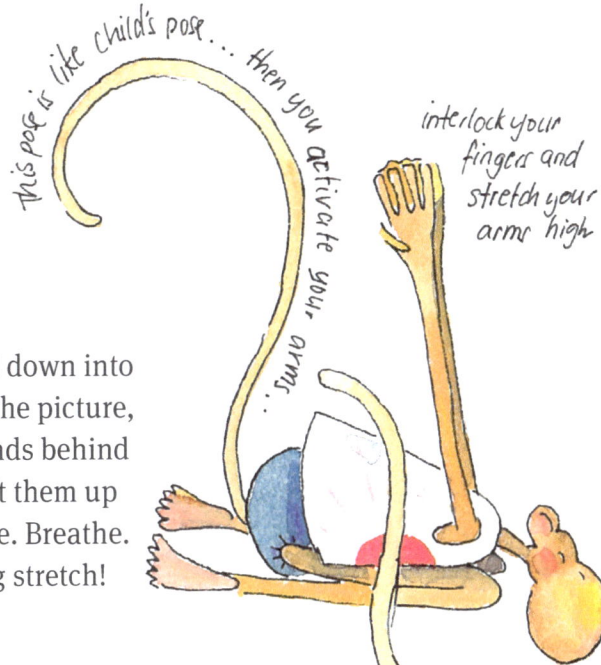

2

Now lift your tailbone and roll onto the crown of your head. Make sure you don't twist your neck in either direction.

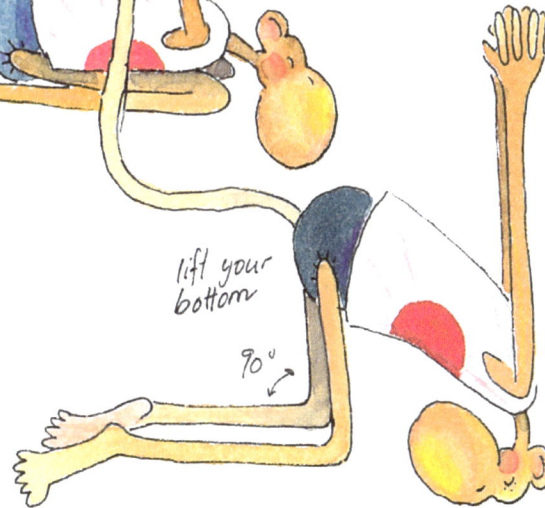

lift your bottom

90°

come onto the crown of your head

stretch those arms high

balance the weight between the head and knees...

BREATHE...

toes can be tucked under!

3

Your legs should be hip-width apart so you are able to look out between the legs. Smile. Take a few breaths and balance the weight on your head and your knees. Stretch your arms high. Breathe and then come into child's pose.

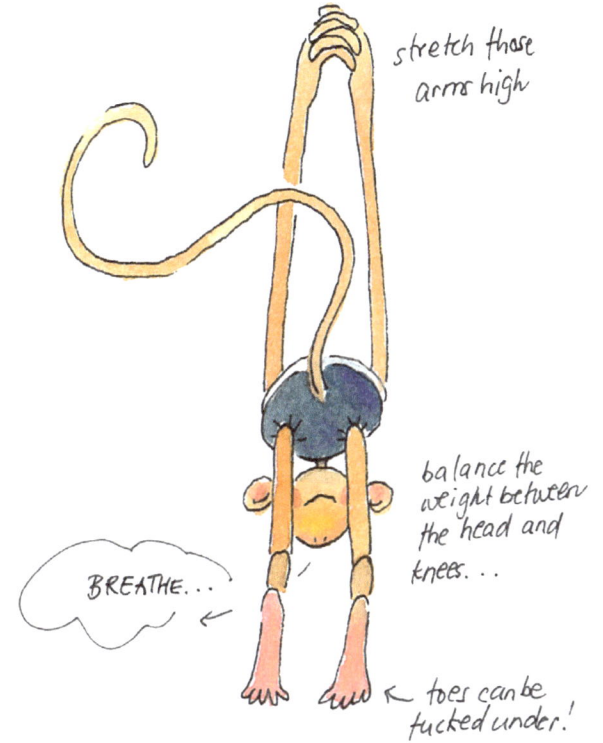

fish pose

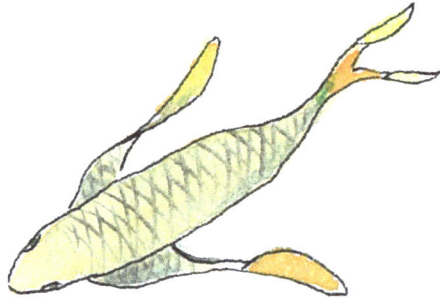

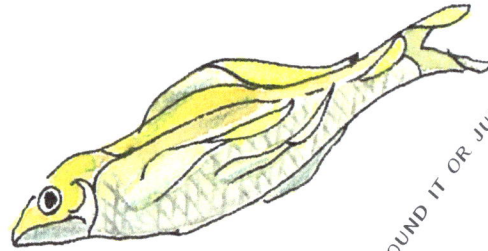

BE LIKE WATER GOING WITH THE FLOW. WHEN THE BOULDER GETS IN THE WAY, OR A BIG ROCK, TRAVEL AROUND IT OR JUMP OVER IT, SWIFT AS A FISH...

TRY TO USE YOUR IMAGINATION WHEN YOU HIT A WALL. THERE ARE WAYS AROUND IT

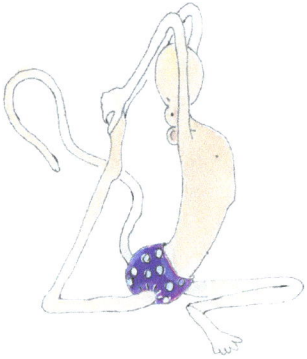

...OR OVER IT!

1

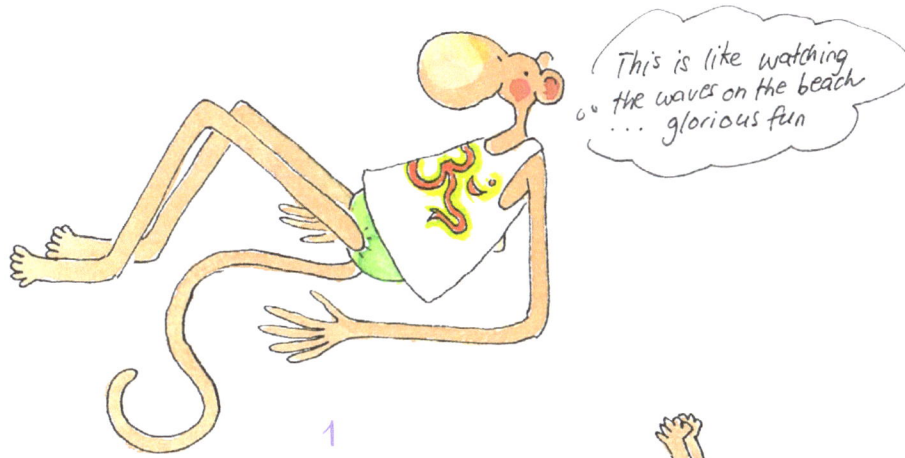

Come onto your elbows as if you are sunbathing or gazing around on the beach.

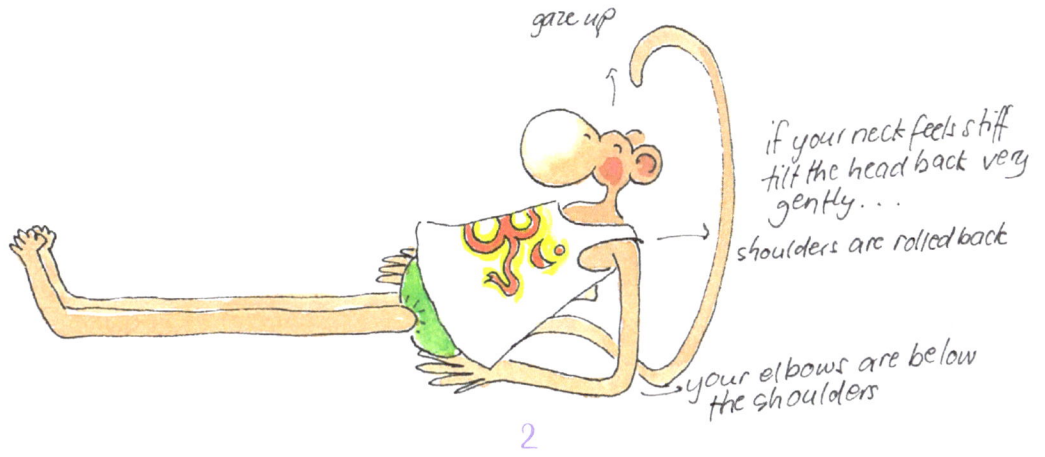

This is like watching the waves on the beach ... glorious fun

gaze up

if your neck feels stiff tilt the head back very gently...

shoulders are rolled back

your elbows are below the shoulders

2

Now slip your hands underneath your lower back and stretch your legs.

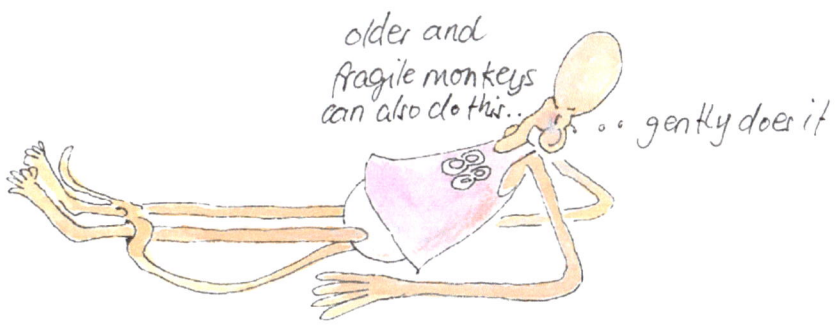

older and fragile monkeys can also do this...

...gently does it

(old monkeys have to be a little careful when trying this pose)

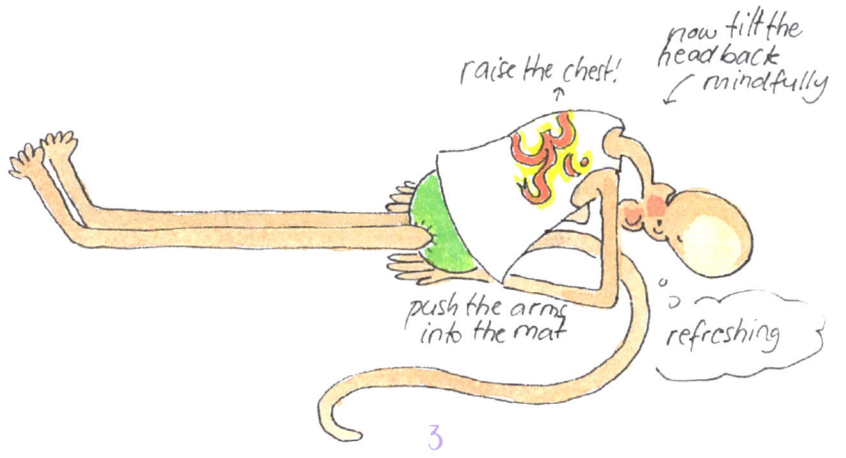

raise the chest!

now tilt the head back mindfully

push the arms into the mat

refreshing

3

Gently (if you can) let your head tilt back. See if the crown of your head reaches the mat. Keep lifting your chest up. Breathe...and count to 20.

happy-baby pose

This is a great hip and leg stretch and generally brings
strength to the belly and makes the back elastic.

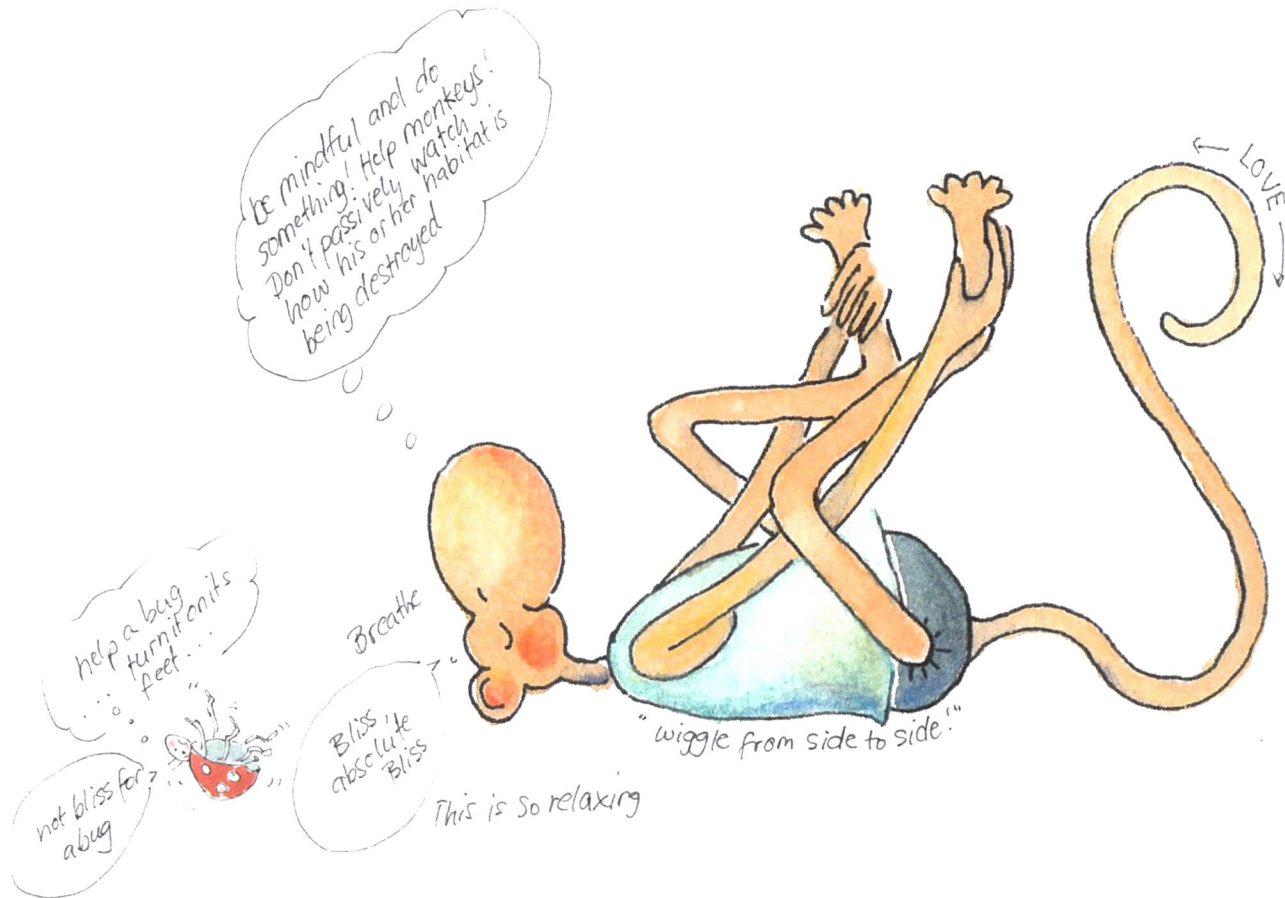

be mindful and do something! Help monkeys! Don't passively watch how his or her habitat is being destroyed

← LOVE →

help a bug turn if on its feet...

not bliss for a bug

Breathe

Bliss absolute Bliss

This is so relaxing

"wiggle from side to side."

Lie flat on your back with your legs bent like an upside-down bug.
Now flip your feet in the direction of your head.
Keep your elbows between your knees. Grab the outside of your feet.
Relax and wiggle about. "Haaaaaaaaaaaaaaaaaaa!"

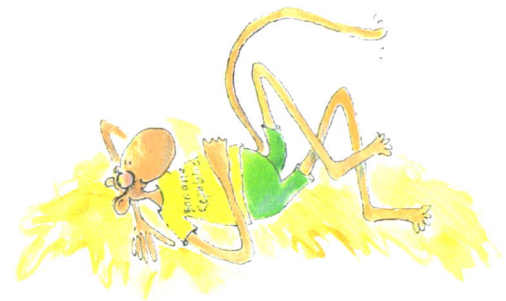

final relaxation

After a balanced practice, even just a 10-minute one, final relaxation gives the body the important chance to regroup and reset itself. It helps you focus and concentrate better as the deepest muscles are given a chance to relax. Never leave a yoga practice without relaxing at the end. Do this for at least 5 minutes.

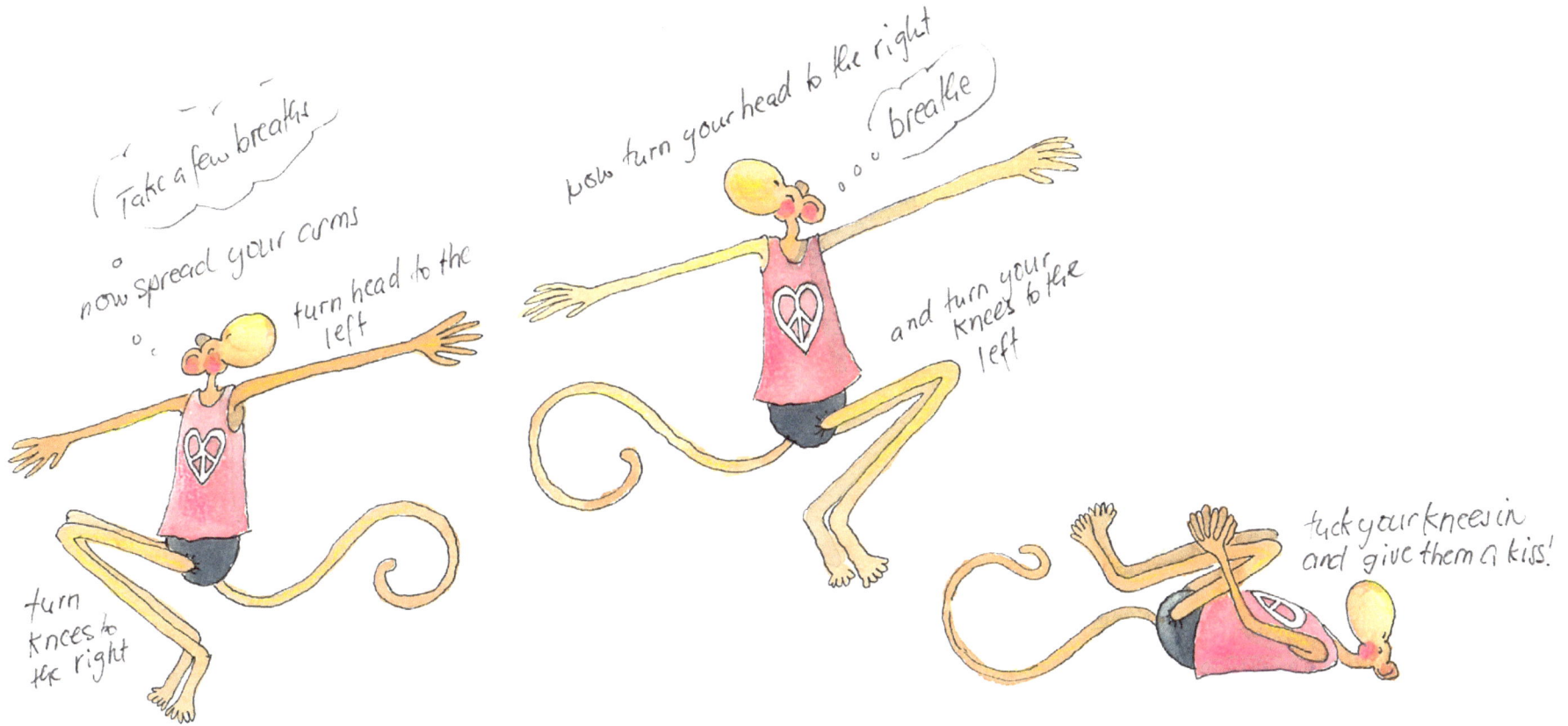

Take a few breaths

now spread your arms

turn head to the left

turn knees to the right

now turn your head to the right

breathe

and turn your knees to the left

tuck your knees in and give them a kiss!

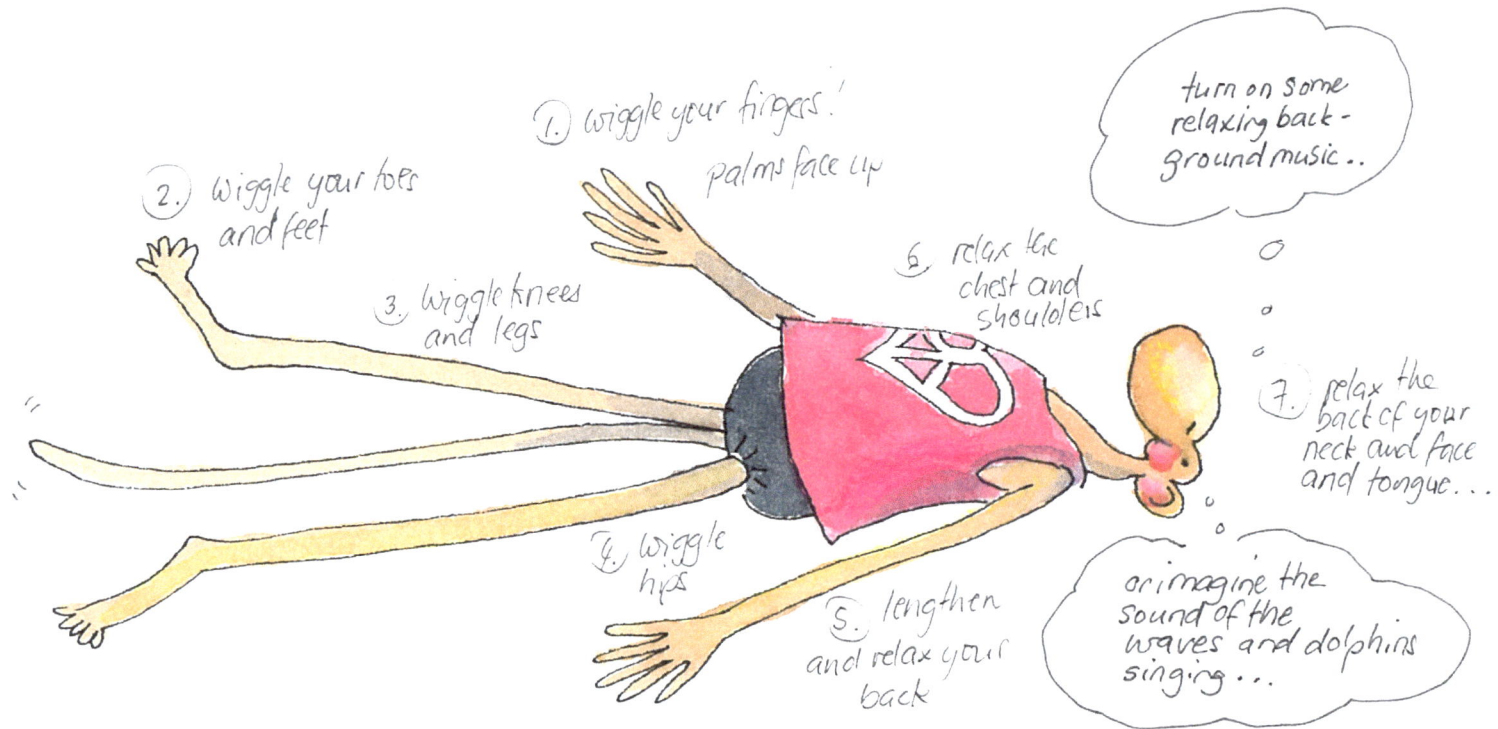

Gently wiggle your toes and fingers and relax
your hips, shoulders and neck. Relax your whole
body and breathe naturally. Stay in relaxation
for a good 5 to 10 minutes. Cover yourself with a
blanket if need be.

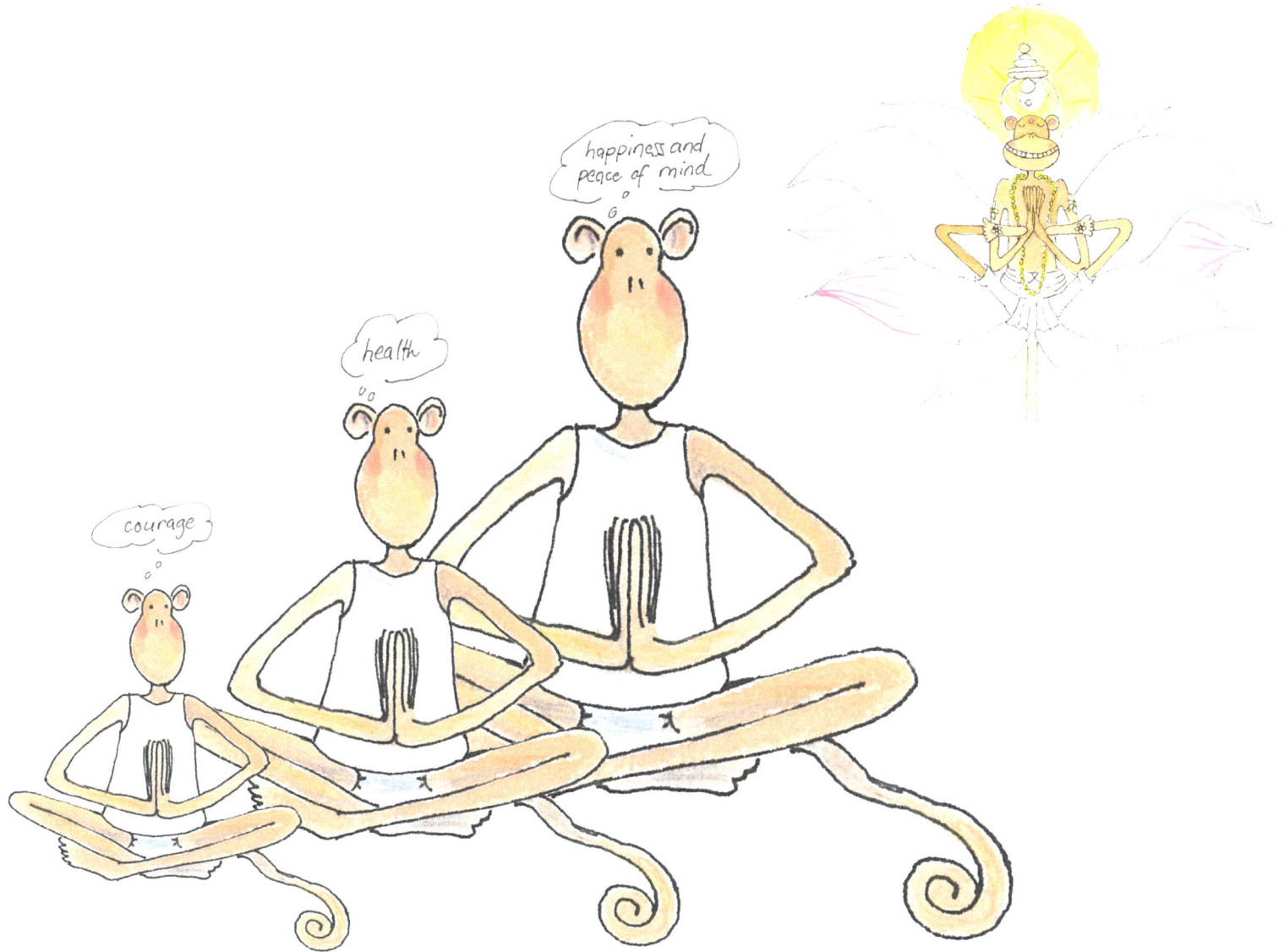

MAKE A WISH FOR PEACE...

NOW CHANT PEACE 3 TIMES AND VISUALISE
NATURE PROSPERING...

BREATHE AND LIVE THE ROCK 'N' ROLL OF UNCONDITIONAL LOVE

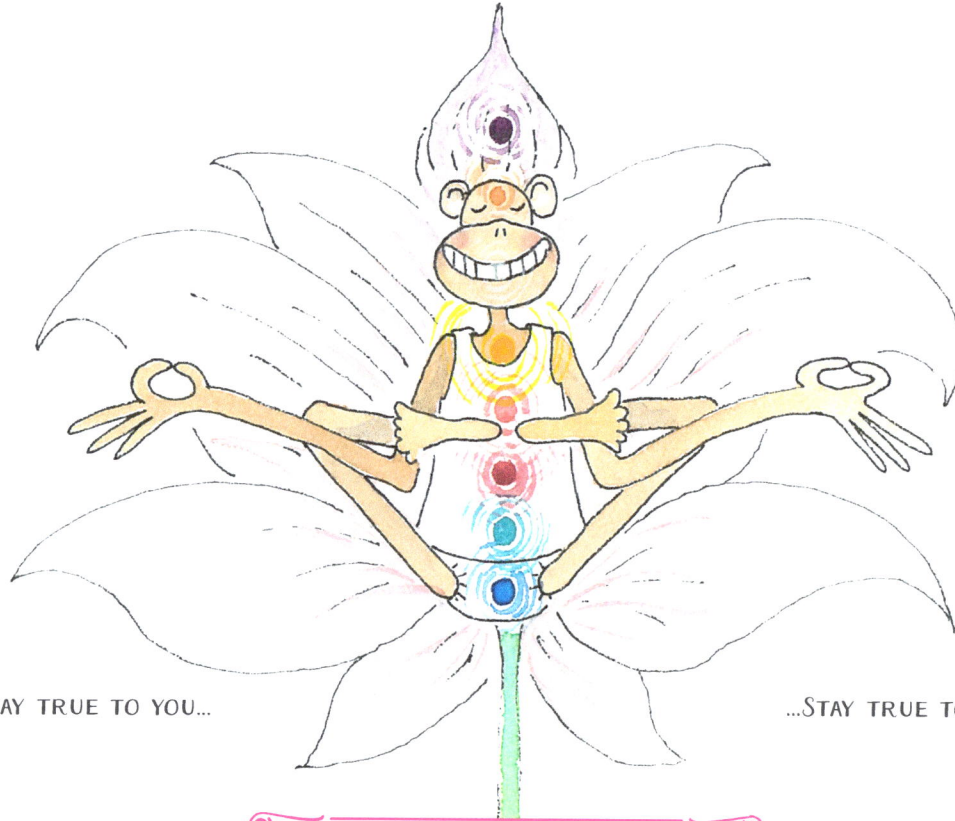

...STAY TRUE TO YOU...   ...STAY TRUE TO YOU...

ZEN POINT

THOSE WHO DON'T FEEL THIS LOVE,
THOSE WHO DON'T DRINK DAWN LIKE
A CUP OF SPRING WATER OR TAKE IN
SUNSET LIKE SUPPER, THOSE WHO
DON'T WANT TO CHANGE, LET THEM
SLEEP...SLEEP...

– RUMI, THE ILLUMINATED RUMI

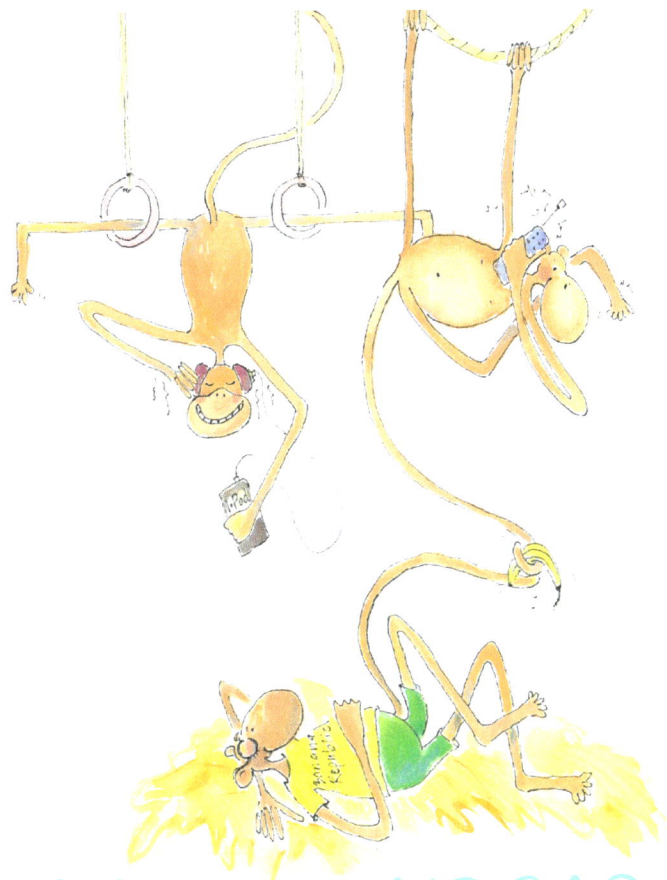

WHAT IS YOGA?

Let's try and explain a bit more what yoga is all about. Have you ever heard of such a thing as "the monkey mind"? Well, if you haven't, neither has Aristotle and he is a monkey.

The monkey mind is the busy "me, me, me," voice in our heads which constantly jumps from one idea to the next and finds it hard to settle on one thing at a time. The mind can easily get distracted by hundreds of other thoughts.

When the monkey mind controls us, we can't concentrate because the thoughts in our heads are like unruly, cheeky monkeys playing havoc with us. If you observe those cheeky monkeys at the zoo you'll see exactly what that's about.

To bring the monkey mind under control, to tame those monkey thoughts in your head, takes concentration, discipline and self- control. Really, in the end, the only one who can be in control of your mind is you.

Now the yogic sages (enlightened, holy masters) have taught for thousands of years that only when the mind, body and soul are in balance and harmony will you understand yourself better.

When you're in comfortable control of your mind and emotions, you won't feel like wanting to control everything else so much and you'll experience a sense of freedom which is invigorating beyond explanation. The sages call this union with your true self.

Wow! Pretty amazing.

By trying to keep focused on the yoga exercises in the previous pages, your mind will begin to become more attuned and clear. You'll start to flow more with your breath, aware of your needs, wishes and personal comfort zone. Everyone is different, and that's a great thing.

Having someone who is familiar with yoga to practice with can help you gain quicker physical control about which way to experience the poses and it's nice to have company.

A sensible teacher can help guide you on your journey, but it is you who knows best how to listen to your inner teacher. This is the beginning of inner freedom. This is what's called meditation or mindfulness.

Mindfulness is the opposite of a full mind. Mindfulness is listening to the quiet voice within your heart and getting to understand the true meaning of: "Who am I truly?" "How can I make this world a better place?"

Have the courage to live your truth, and when you make mistakes along the way, have the creativity to get back on your bike and be the change you wish to see in this world.

THE INs AND OUTs OF BREATH

Breathing not only keeps you alive, it makes you feel alive. If we breathe properly our life force is activated. The life force is the force that makes you get out of bed and helps you keep going throughout the day. Breath is a bit like a best friend, it inspires, it gives you energy and enlivens the body.

Running, swimming and exercising activate breathing. When your breath is activated and you breathe more deeply, more oxygen is pumped through the blood. Fresh blood flow helps you think better and concentrate longer and makes you feel calmer and more positive.

In yoga breathing is very important. When we concentrate we tend to forget to breathe or breathe only very shallowly. So, when you practice a new pose or a pose which is challenging, watch that you don't forget to breathe. Generally, you'll find yourself breathing in as you stretch the body upward and breathing out as you bend downward. It's the natural way. While holding a pose you breathe in and out several times.

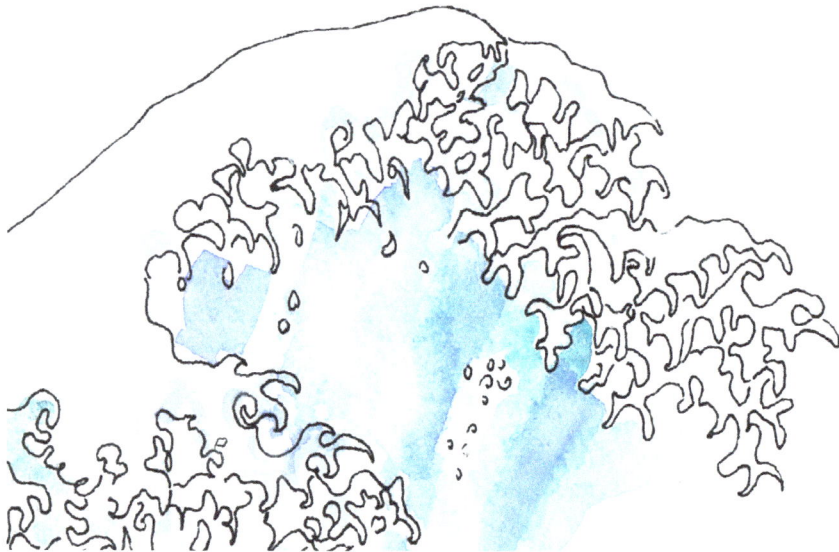

If we don't move enough or stay inactive for too long our breathing suffers as well. We become lethargic and sickly. Yoga increases the quality of breathing and can help those who suffer from asthma, allergies and feelings of depression. Breathing is great for the imagination. It's literally inspiring in so many ways.

One in and out breath is counted as one breath. We tend to count the time we stay in a pose by breaths. So, for example, we stay in a pose for 3 to 5 or even 10 breaths. Smaller children are encouraged to count to 5 or 10 while in a pose—they do not count breaths; a gentle reminder—not to forget to breathe—is enough. Those who've done yoga for some time and are confident can start concentrating on deep and calm breathing through the nose. As long as we remember to breathe, that is important.

The quality of air is also important. We live in a world where the air is often polluted. Even the astronauts can see a grey layer of pollution from space now. That is very sad as it means our planet has difficulty with all the pollution and not only humans but plants, animals and the earth's surface are equally suffering. We can make this world a better place by keeping the air we breathe clean, the rivers pure and our hearts open. You're not separate from any other living and breathing beings. It's important to understand that. Whatever we do (or don't do) has an effect on others too. Keeping your body healthy and giving it what it needs helps you be a more mindful person for this planet.

Go to a park or somewhere where the air is fresh and breathe deeply. Think of ways you can help keep our planet healthy and the air clean. Try not to be greedy. Keep pollution down. Yoga helps you keep the body healthy and the lungs strong, but at the same time we need to think of ways not to pollute this beautiful world.

Have the courage and imagination to follow your dreams. Everything is connected in our world. The air which enters our lungs goes back out into the world again. We all breathe the very same air.

Without air, we couldn't live longer than a few minutes. Breathe! Think of your breath as your friend.

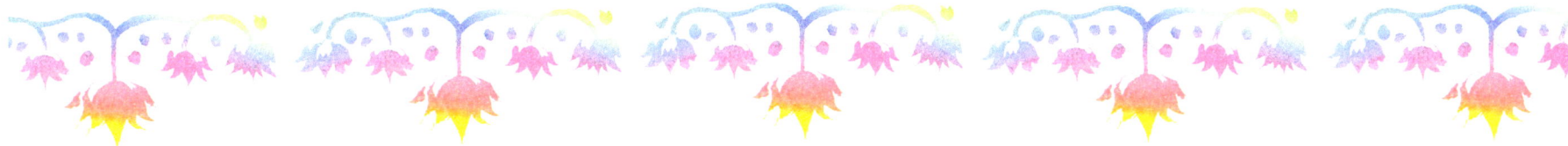

To Happiness, Health and Courage!

"One must confront vague ideas with clear images." Jean Luc Goddard

To all who wish to take responsibility for their own well-being, and who care about the wellness of their fellow human beings:

The author/illustrator of this book, Bibi, doesn't advocate any particular health program, but believes that the ancient art/science of Hatha Yoga presented here ought to be available to every person concerned with maintaining and/or improving their own health. Yoga is a health tool which is life-enhancing and restorative. It counteracts the stressful and unbalanced elements and demands in our life. It is complementary to sports, the creative arts and good nutrition, among other things, and is meant for parents, children, office workers, labourers, intellectuals, the poor and the rich, by complimenting both modern and holistic health methods.

The person practicing yoga should use their own judgment, or consult their physician or holistic health-care professional for any specific solutions regarding their individual concerns.

Yoga is not a substitute cure for serious illnesses. However, it can serve as a preventive before serious illness occurs.

Hatha yoga is one of the most ancient tools supporting those who believe in taking responsibility for their own well-being, as well as that of their fellow human beings.

About Bibi and Her Kids' Yoga Pioneering Years

Bibi is a trained primary school teacher with a post-graduate degree in Theatre and an honours degree in Literary Translation. She works as a children's book illustrator and writer, among other things. Bibi became a White Lotus Certified Yoga Instructor in 2004.

Having practiced hatha yoga in the UK since 1994 and enjoying its benefits, Bibi felt compelled to bring yoga to the young and curious, so started teaching yoga at Tokyo International School when she was living in Japan. "We used to do yoga on the school roof-top, in the wind and the sun, and sometimes we had to roll up our mats and run inside when the weather became stormy. We became like a small family. The kids loved the final relaxation pose, covered with the fluffy white spotted red blankets, listening to stories about mother nature and dolphins singing in the ocean, with the cooling wind blowing around us. We always had a good mix of boys and girls aged between 5 and 10. The kids were amazed to find out that a hundred years ago, yoga was practiced by males only. It would have been inconceivable that girls, let alone those from other cultures, would practice and eventually teach it."

Bibi brings a sense of wonder and an "all things possible" view to a world that often-times acts impossibly. The fact children saw themselves progress in ways they wouldn't have imagined at first, gave them a lot of self-confidence and made Bibi very proud of them.

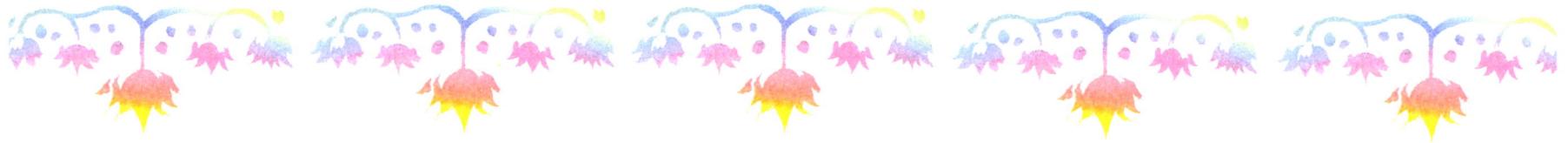

MY GRATITUDE

My mum, a constant supporter of what I do (an admirer because I am her daughter and she thinks she could not do what I do! Typical mum, I love you).

Thank you Myn Whyman, Partick Newell, Nonie Adams, Sue Aspinall, Rachel Dickinson, Ikuyo Maeda, for supporting my idea of bringing yoga and meditation to children in schools and for giving me the opportunity to teach classes at International Schools in Tokyo. Thank you to my instructors and lifelong teacher training friends from the Krishnamacharya lineage T.K.V. Desikachar, Kaustub Desikachar, Ken Bond, Paul Reynolds, Ganga White, Tracey Ritch, Cheri Clampett, Danny Paradise, Pete Humes, Lisa Austin McClintock, Diana Mickey Erkietain, Sada Anand Sing Khalsa, director at Ikoma Mountain Yoga Retreat Center 3HO Japan, and Gurmukh Kaur Khalsa, Legacy Teacher of Kundalini Yoga as taught by Yogi Bhajan.

A special thank you to Osada San for encouraging me to get this book out into the world after the 2011 Japan earthquake and Fukushima nuclear tragedy. (Her father, Dr Orata Osada, who wrote "Children of the A-Bomb", took a deep interest in pedagogy and children's mental and emotional health).

Thank you to all my friends and students who supported me and cheered me on in getting this book out into the world: Anne-Laure Fleuri Winkler, Donna Alley, Stefanie Schuller, Rosmarie and Nobu Nakanishi, Motoko Nakaishi, Uncle Richard and Renata Drtina for the help with edits, Barbara Panettieri for helping translate it into German, Claudia Sanches for translating it into Spanish, to Sarah and Akira for translating it into Japanese, Laurel and Collin Chiles for their love and support at Pinnacle Books, Jane Costello for helping me simplify, Gabi Bliss for her creative inspired lyrics to keep me going, Akiko from Uehara Gallery, Maureen Hudson Nampujinpa, an artist who inspired us all with her strength after the 2011 Japan earthquake, Ogasawara San from Sur Mur Gallery, Koda San and all the staff from Levain Boulangerie Tokyo, Eiji from Kuumba International Tokyo, Karen and Dylan Mc Dermott from Serenity Press for tying up the threads, Lisa Benson and Joanne Fedler for directing me and your support. Thank you to Myrlia Purcell from the NZ Jane Goodall Institute of New Zealand for all her support.

Big thank you to Dr Jane Goodall for endorsing my work and understanding its vision which hopefully will reach people far and wide on many levels.

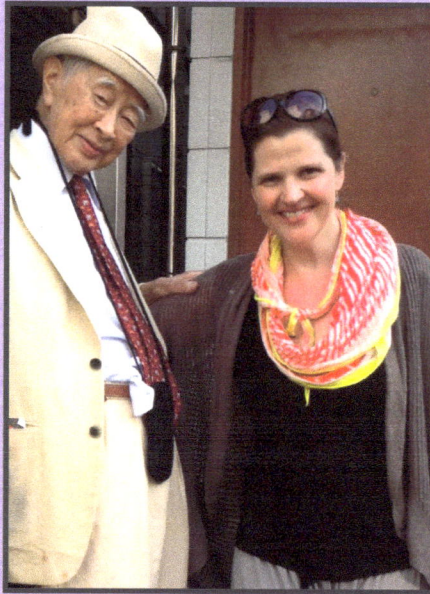

ME AND MY SPECIAL FRIEND
PAUL AKIO SAWADA WHO
STUCK WITH ME
AND THIS PROJECT THROUGH
THICK AND THIN.

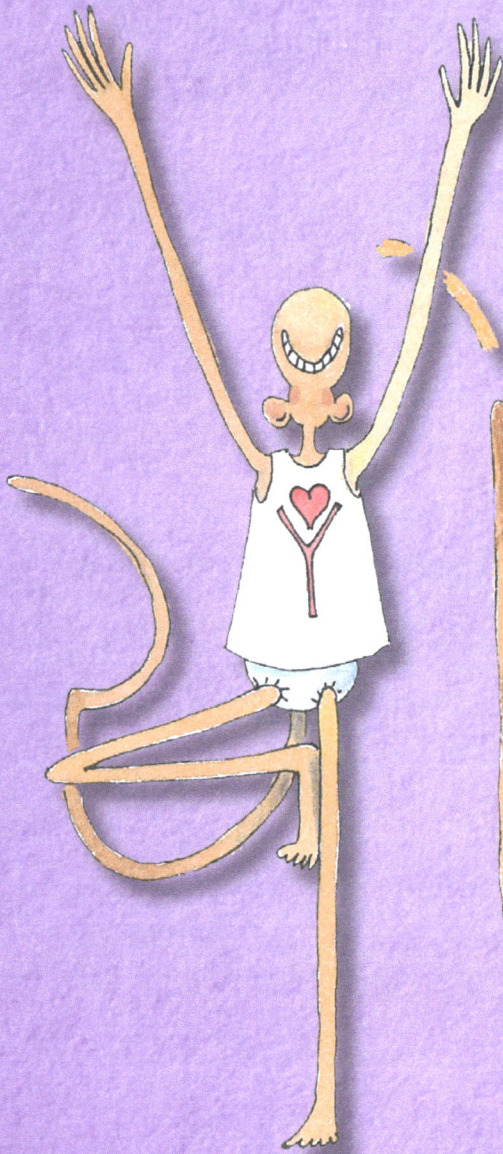

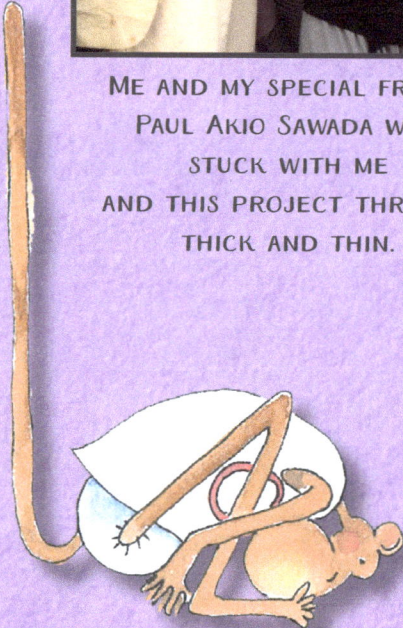

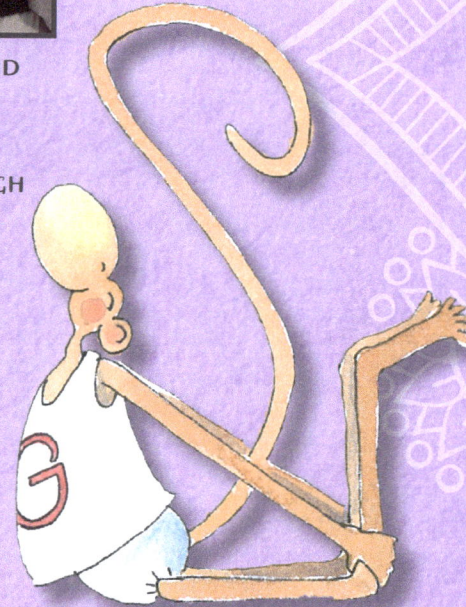

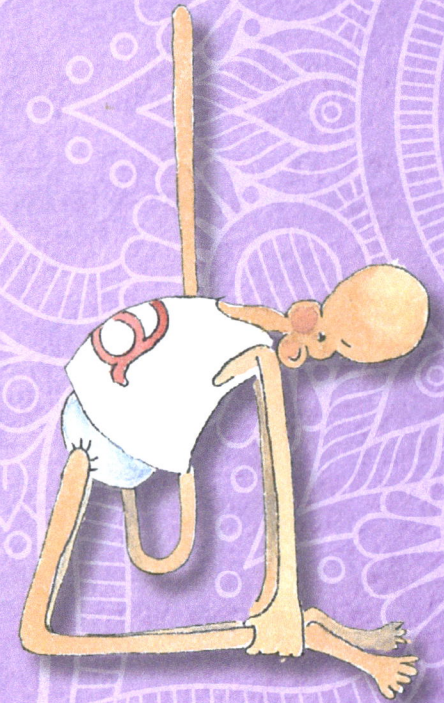

...SEE YOU IN THE NEXT BOOK...

www.ingramcontent.com/pod-product-compliance
Lightning Source LLC
Chambersburg PA
CBHW040711150426

42811CB00061B/1814